·

# Meditating to Attain a Healthy Body Weight

·

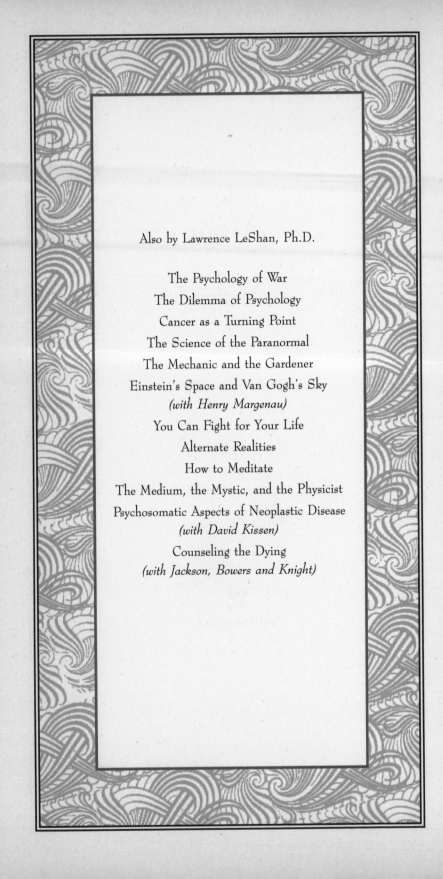

Also by Lawrence LeShan, Ph.D.

# Meditating
## · to ·
## Attain
## · a ·
## Healthy
## Body
## Weight

*Lawrence LeShan, Ph.D.*

BANTAM BOOKS

New York   Toronto
London   Sydney
Auckland

MEDITATING TO ATTAIN A HEALTHY BODY WEIGHT
A BANTAM BOOK
*published in association with Doubleday*

PUBLISHING HISTORY
*Doubleday hardcover edition / June 1994*
*Bantam trade paperback edition / May 1995*

*The Library of Congress has cataloged the hardcover edition
of this book as follows:*
LeShan, Lawrence L., 1920–
Meditating to attain a healthy body weight / Lawrence LeShan.—1st ed.
p.    cm.
1. Reducing.   2. Meditation.   I. Title
RM222.2.L4265   1994
613.2'5—dc20                                                      93-43320
                                                                        CIP

ISBN 0-553-37372-2

*Published simultaneously in the United States and Canada*

---

*Bantam Books are published by Bantam Books, a division of Bantam
Doubleday Dell Publishing Group, Inc. Its trademark, consisting of the
words "Bantam Books" and the portrayal of a rooster, is Registered in U.S.
Patent and Trademark Office and in other countries. Marca Registrada.
Bantam Books, 1540 Broadway, New York, New York 10036.*

---

PRINTED IN THE UNITED STATES OF AMERICA

BVG      0 9 8 7 6 5 4 3 2 1

*This book is dedicated to Eda LeShan,*
*who taught me to understand*
*the courage and dignity*
*we human beings show in our search*
*for health and growth.*

# Contents

·

•

Meditating to Attain a Healthy Body Weight

•

# Introducing the Author

·

When Larry's editor asked for an introduction to this book, describing his background and explaining how he became involved with this subject, the task, perhaps naturally enough, fell to me.

While meditation and diet may at first seem rather separate disciplines, they do, in fact, connect in a way that has been a focus of his work as a psychologist for many years—making the link between mind and body in pursuit of health.

As long ago as 1950 a colleague, Dick Worthington, reported to Larry that while giving a psychological diagnostic test to a great many subjects, he had found himself able to see some similarities among people with cancer. The two men felt this was a clue worth following.

Working with cancer patients who had been diagnosed as hopeless and near death, Larry began to try to develop a special kind of psychotherapy that might be helpful. (He realized later that he was trying to reinforce the immune system, whose function was understood only after his work had begun.)

Fifteen or twenty years later, a whole new area of psychology had developed in this field, and Larry's interest in the link between mind and body took him in another direction—exploring ESP, parapsychology, and psychic healing.

After absorbing as much as he could of written reports, he came to believe that extraordinary mental activities do really happen. These occur when an individual or a group enters a specific state of consciousness that sometimes causes remarkable paranormal events. Often this state of consciousness is learned through intensive training in meditation. He studied the major religious mystics and clairvoyants and analyzed their descriptions of entering an "alternate reality." He was surprised to discover that physicists described a reality entirely in agreement.

Over the course of several years, he trained himself through a series of meditation exercises, to enter an alternate state of consciousness required for parapsychologial events to take place. Instead of trying to learn how to predict the future, or guess at cards, he felt that there was one aspect of this work in alternate realities which could be useful: psychic healing. By pursuing some experiments on his own (and some with our daughter and me as early subjects) he felt psychic healing could be a useful psychic tool. On a bus to a demonstration in Washington against the Vietnam War, he "healed" his daughter's burned and badly swollen fingers; in California, when I slammed the trunk of the car on my hand, we figured we needed to go to a hospital where I might have permanent loss of fingers—so why not try this new tool he'd been practicing. After a few minutes of psychic healing I regained the full use of my hand without pain. There were, soon, hundreds of stories, all carefully documented; Larry had not joined "the crazies," "the flakeheads." He insisted on the most rigorous study and experimentation. There are now several books dealing with this work.

Eventually he decided psychic healing could probably be taught to others by intensive work with specific, carefully selected meditations. Very much of a skeptic, I decided to attend one of his early seminars in order to try to understand what he was doing. That workshop forever changed my life. Having always lived in "the here and now," I found myself capable of living in a different reality. Raised as a practical agnostic, I now accept everyday reality as one of many myths. I can meditate; I can even heal on occasion.

Psychic healing and meditation remain an area for continuing growth and development. Several years ago we both came to the conclusion that learning to meditate—to use one's consciousness in new ways—could be helpful in dealing with many problems, and that there might be specific meditations that could help people deal with many of the challenges, which, in daily life, they could not seem to solve. The meditations and exercises described in this book (tested by himself and others, to his satisfaction—and he is a tough taskmaster) have proved to be helpful to many people who have otherwise been unable to lose weight.

*Eda LeShan*
*Fall 1993*

# · 1 ·

≋

## Meditating for a
## Healthy Body Weight

ENRY WAS A thirty-nine-year-old lawyer and had been overweight except for brief periods most of his adult life. He had tried all the major diets and lost some weight with most of them, but it returned fairly quickly. He had attended group meetings and twice gone for several weeks to residential centers for specialized diet work, again had lost weight and seen it return within a few months. On his fortieth birthday he came to see me to work out a meditation program to help him with what had become a serious health problem.

Henry expected me to give him a simple meditation that was already designed for weight loss—sort of like taking a suit of clothes off the rack or going to the druggist for a headache pill. As we talked he realized that if such a thing existed—one mental pill that would work for everyone—he would have found it long before. We talked about the fact that a realistic program would have to be more complex than this and also one that was designed for him, not one that was exactly the same for everybody. Together we designed a four-part program that would help him to lose weight and keep it off—a program built on what we have learned from two thousand years of experience with meditation and from a hundred years of experience with the scientific understanding of the human mind and how to use it in ways that best achieve our goals. This book is about how that program can be used by others to design their own weight loss programs.

The four parts of Henry's program started with meditations designed to strengthen the ability of his mind to cope with problems and to increase his confidence in his ability to cope and deal effectively with difficulties and temptations. An athlete who is going to compete in a particular event first tunes and trains his body generally and in an overall sense before he starts the specific training, for example, pole vaulting and running the marathon.

The second part of the program was designed specifically to help him lose weight, to help him reach what for him as a unique individual would be a healthy body weight. This, to continue the analogy of the athlete, is the specific training for the athletic event.

The third part of the program comprised a group of meditations for the particularly hard and discouraging times that come during any serious attempt we human beings make to change. What do we do when the going gets very rough and we feel we are failing, our resolve and energy diminishing? This part of the program was designed for those times.

The fourth part consisted of a series of exercises in which Henry would look at his life in a very realistic and tough manner and find ways to get more joy and zest out of it. After all, if he was going to give up some of the pleasure of food, he would need more, and more realistic, pleasures to take its place. What, realistically, would be more rewarding to this unique person—Henry—than his present patterns of action? How could he determine these rewards and move toward them?

Henry found that he could work at this individually designed program and that he was able to stay with it. He lost the amount of weight necessary to feel good about himself. In the years since, he has—with a few pounds of variation each way—held his new weight. He feels good about his life and is enjoying it.

⌒

HELEN WAS VERY eager to lose fifteen pounds and keep them off. On one diet or another she had managed to lose that much weight, but it always returned over the next year. When she was thinner she felt better and healthier, believed that she looked better, but within a relatively short time she regained what she had lost.

After a discussion of the possibilities and problems of using meditation as a way of helping herself deal with the problem, Helen resolved to try once again. She decided on one thirty-minute session a day, five days a week. She felt that her weekends were so disorganized and hectic that trying to meditate on Saturday and Sunday would probably wreck the entire program. For the first track—the general discipline approach—she chose a breath-counting meditation for fifteen minutes. For the second track she chose, also for fifteen minutes, a Thousand Petal Lotus meditation with the word "hungry" as the center. In addition, for one meal every other day, she ate in silence while she "one-pointed" her food. (The details of these meditation techniques will be described in Chapters 2 and 3).

All went well for several weeks, during which time Helen found that she was eating less and simply feeling hungry less of the time. Then she underwent a period of stress in her work and began to be very hungry and "binge" from time to time. She chose, in addition to her regular program, to add a mantra for an extra fifteen minutes on the five weekdays. A mantra is a phrase repeated over and over again while focusing on it and nothing else as completely as possible. The mantra she chose was "I am in charge of my life." About two weeks later, she realized that her weight loss program seemed to be back on line and functioning. She kept using the mantra, as well as her original chosen group.

She had decided originally on a six-week program. At the end of that time she carefully thought about her experience and decided to continue the same program, except that she would change the "center" of her Thousand Petal Lotus meditation to "food." She continued this program for another six weeks and then another six. She then felt that not only had she lost the weight she wanted to, but she also felt confident about keeping it off. Somehow food no longer seemed a problem area. She then decided to enter the next stage of the program and use it to try to increase her zest and enthusiasm for life generally—to find new ways of increasing her enjoyment of her life and ways to get more out of the things she had enjoyed before. She started with two exercises described in Chapter 7, the Every Wednesday (page 103) and the Overnight Miracle (page 108) techniques. From these, over a period of time, she went on to others.

At the end of the first year, she has kept her weight down and reports that her life is busy and zestful. She is looking forward to new adventures.

~

Marvin had been grossly overweight since childhood. When he decided to try meditation, he weighed 405 pounds, was five feet five inches tall, and twenty-eight years old. Although strong psychological forces in his childhood had played a part in his original overeating, intensive psychotherapy as an adult had not succeeded in resolving the problem. The dieting organizations and groups he had joined had provided only temporary help. A long stay at a residential diet center took off about half the weight he needed to lose, but that had returned within a one-year period. He hated himself, felt very bad when he had to squeeze past people in a crowded bus or movie, and each time he felt these bad feelings, he seemed to try to comfort himself with food. His physician repeatedly told him that he had to lose well over 150 pounds or face serious medical consequences, but he was unable to do so. Finally as a last resort, he decided to try the meditation approach. He discussed this with his physician, who agreed that it was worth trying and said that she would give him regular medical examinations during the process.

After several discussions of the resources and the problems involved in this approach, he chose a program of forty minutes a day, every day, on awakening. For the general meditation work, he chose a meditation in which he would concentrate on visualizing a spot of light slowly traveling in a definite path around his body, from the right fingertip, down around each leg, out to the left fingertip and over the head to the point of origin. He would do this fifteen minutes a day. He would also "breath-count" for another ten minutes. For the specific meditations on losing weight, he chose one in which he concentrated on which part of his body he "felt" hunger in, and used a special technique (see Chapter 3 for details) to drain the tension out of this area. In addition, he decided to do a five-minute "centering" meditation before each meal and to eat one meal a day in silence and "one-pointing" (trying to be aware of one thing and nothing else) the sensations in his mouth as he ate.

The program seemed to be helping for nearly a month. During that time he was generally less hungry and "binged" only twice. Then he began to feel increasing tension and an increasing desire to eat. He added to his program an intensive meditation called Safe Harbor (described in detail in

Chapter 4). After about a week of this, the extra tension seemed to diminish and his weight loss program was back on line.

He continued this work for a year, reevaluating the details of the program every five weeks, but—since it seemed to him to be effective—making only minor changes. At the end of that time, he began to do some of the exercises described in Chapter 6 to learn what ways he could find to get more fun and zest out of his life. He is still very overweight for his age, but he feels more comfortable, is beginning to enjoy exercising in a gymnasium, and is no longer self-conscious when he goes out in public. His physician is very pleased, but still makes it clear Marvin has a long way to go.

ALL THROUGH HUMAN history there have been people who tried to find ways to develop their minds and bring themselves closer to their potential. They tried to deal with their minds as an athlete deals with his or her body, so that they could roam more freely and completely through reality and live with more zest and joy. Wherever and whenever they were—whether in India six centuries before Christ, during the Greek and Roman Classical period, in medieval monasteries, in twelfth-century Spain, or in eighteenth-century Poland and Russia, the methods they developed independently were very similar. We call these methods "meditations." Their goal is to enable you to get more out of life and to move more completely in whatever directions you choose.

A meditation is a specialized tool for affecting one's own mind and personality. In a gymnasium there are special tools for affecting the body—exercise machines of various kinds, weights, running tracks, etc. These affect the body in different ways—some strengthen the muscles more, some strengthen the heart and lung system, and so forth. Similarly meditations affect you in different ways. They should be carefully chosen in terms of who you are and what you want to do. Where, when, and how you meditate will vary. There is no right way for everyone. Just as there is no one medical prescription that cures all diseases in all people, there is no one meditation that solves all problems for everyone.

Similarly there is no ideal weight that applies to all people of specific heights and sex. We have different bone structures, types of body build, endocrine and digestive systems, and different everything else. We are accustomed to this fact when we talk about fingerprints, but most people feel that in all other aspects, specific rules should apply to everyone.

One aspect of this is the fact that it is far more difficult for some people to lose weight than it is for others. We know today that heredity plays a major part in how your body uses the food you eat. On exactly the same diet, the same amount of exercise, and the same number of calories, some people will gain weight, others hold steady, and still others lose. There appear to be complex, little understood patterns in your genes that determine how your body will react. This is one of the reasons no one diet applies to everyone.

Your goal weight should not be determined by the advertisements you see on television and in the magazines. Not everyone should be pencil thin and have a twenty-two-inch waist. This may be the goal of a model who wants to appear on the cover of *Vogue,* but you should aim for a weight that makes you comfortable, that keeps your physician from focusing on weight every time you come into the office, and that allows you reasonable (for your age) movement and athletic activities. I stress this point because we live in an age in which advertising makes us more and more uncomfortable about our weight in order to sell new goods and services, and in which the pressure has grown so great that children in elementary and high school classes are developing eating disorders in their attempts to become thin enough to feel attractive. If you believe that by looking like a refugee from Somalia you will be beautiful and will feel good about yourself, you need a psychiatrist, not a method of moving toward the right weight for you.

Each of the four parts of the weight control program in this book will be described in detail in a chapter of its own. However, before we get into these particulars, let me make some general comments about the process of meditation.

How much time should you take to meditate each day? You must choose this yourself. I would suggest something like a half-hour a day to start. But be realistic. If you will not do this (and you know yourself very well), then choose an amount of time you will be able to do. I might wish, for example, that I were the kind of person who would give this an hour a day. But I am not and I know it, so if I choose this much time, in a week I will begin to skimp the periods (promising myself to make it up the next day) and then to skip days from time to time (promising myself that I will do twice as much the next day), and as a result, in two weeks I will owe myself ten hours and the whole program will have gone down the drain. I choose the amount of time I will be able to do and then I make a commitment and a promise to myself. And I do everything I can to keep it!

Most of us are pretty good at keeping promises to others and pretty bad at keeping promises to ourselves. One of the goals of meditation is to learn to treat yourself as a serious person, a person to be protected and well taken care of. This involves keeping your promises to yourself.

For example, there will be days when you simply have not been able to find the time to meditate. Unexpected emergencies filled the time you usually use, and the rest of the day was spent dealing with one problem after another. It is now midnight and you are exhausted. You are tempted to say to yourself that there is no point in trying to meditate when you are so tired, that you will clearly get nothing out of it, and that the intelligent thing would be to do twice as much tomorrow. This "twelve o'clock blues" is one of the commonest traps on the meditation road. If you fall into it, the same kind of thing will happen over and over again, and eventually you will realize that you have abandoned the entire program. The thing to do is to do the meditation in spite of how tired you are.

Very often these will turn out to be the most fulfilling sessions. And also, if you do this a few times, you will miraculously begin to find time to meditate during the day. The time will "appear."

Where and when do you meditate? Surely it is helpful if you do it at the same time and in the same place every day. It is nice to have a special time and a place with "good vibes" to work in, but that may not be possible for you, and it is not strictly necessary. Pick a time and place when and where you are most likely to be free of interruption. If your schedule is such that it has to be different places and times on different days, go ahead. Anything that is so precious and fragile it can be done only under ideal conditions probably is not worth very much anyhow. However, it is nice to have conditions as close as possible to ideal, so give some thought to where and when and do your best.

How do you know when the time is up? Suppose you have decided on fifteen minutes for this particular meditation and your eyes are closed as you do it. How do you know when the fifteen minutes are up? The answer is simple—you cheat. Put a clock or watch with a readable face directly in front of you, but far enough away so that you can see it at a glance and still not be bothered or distracted by the ticking. From time to time, as you are dealing with one distraction or another, look at it. After a while you won't have to do this very often. You will get so accurate that you will know pretty well when the time is up and will have to glance at the clock only once. Another possibility is to get some sort of soft alarm like an egg timer perhaps, or a muffled alarm clock. Set it and get on with your business.

Once we have set up a program for a specific meditation, we do not skip or skimp it. But what about doing it for a *longer* period if we feel like it on a specific occasion? This is legitimate, but do not overdo it. Like salt in your food, a certain amount of meditation in your life can be positive and helpful. Too much is not. One can have too much of anything!

In the early days of psychotherapy this was not understood and very often a psychotherapy hour would be scheduled for five or six times a week. This certainly increased the therapist's income, but it tended to have a negative effect on the recovery process of the patient. For one thing, life often began to center around the therapy instead of the other way round. Patients often found it more and more difficult, for example, to make decisions on their own without first "talking it over with my shrink"! Psychotherapy and meditation are development programs whose purpose is to increase the zest, color, and validity of daily life, not to replace it. So increase the time of one or another meditation if you feel like it, but do not put too much of it into your life nor too much salt into your food. People differ so much, it is not really possible to make any rules about how much is too much, but so far as this is possible, I would say that if you are meditating more than two hours a day you had better take a good look at the rest of your life and find out why you are giving away so much time from it. Even the most orthodox and old-line psychoanalyst would not recommend more than two hours a day of psychotherapy. There are real limits to the speed of growth; a baby takes nine months and an oak tree twenty years, and you are not going to be able to speed up these processes. I once knew a very intelligent man who decided to try to grow and change through meditation. He took a three-year period and meditated six hours a day, six days a week. At the end of that time the only change in him we could observe was that he was three years older.

Going away for a special seminar or retreat is, of course, something else. We may work very intensively during these special times. In the East this is called "going to the mountain." You go away for a limited period in order to change yourself and to work in new ways and to find new ways in which to continue your work when you return. In Western development theory and schools we go to the mountain in order to return to everyday life and the marketplace. That is where we live—and hopefully live much better because of the intensive work we did on the mountain and the work we do on ourselves while we are living our lives in the outside world.

All the meditations in this book are tried and true. That is to say they have been tested on a large number of people and each one was very good for some of them, fairly good for others, not very good for some, and completely irrelevant for some others. This is true for all methods of growth from specific types of psychotherapy to the various disciplines and art forms, and to the specific forms of meditation.

All the meditations presented here are guaranteed. The guarantee is that when you work with them the things that happen when people work with meditation will happen. This, of course, includes nothing much happening!

Do you need to meditate in a special position—an Eastern lotus position with your legs interlocked, or sitting with a straight spine in a chair, or anything like this? Different schools of meditation have recommended different positions, and there has been absolutely no agreement. About all they do agree on is that if you have been trained to be in any position to the degree that you get the least discomfort and the fewest signals from your body that you are cramped, use that one. We Westerners are most comfortable in an armchair or perhaps, for the younger of us, lying on the floor. Use one of these. You can also do it lying in bed, but you will have to fight extra hard to keep from falling asleep.

Whichever position you use, falling asleep will be one of the likely results. Our minds resist meditation, resist the discipline of it, and the most common way of expressing that resistance is to go to sleep. All you can do is to be aware of this, to try not to, and—if it happens—resolve to try harder not to do it the next time.

And as we are on the subject of the difficulties of meditation, it is important that you be aware of one thing: nobody learns to meditate well! Practice with any of the meditations presented in this book as long and as hard as you wish, you will still have frequent distractions, wanderings off, going blank, etc. As you practice, what will happen is that your meditation sessions will get more erratic—some of them "very good," in the sense that there were long periods when you were involved with them, doing just them, awake and alert, before you drifted off again. Then there will be others in which your mind seems to be like a herd of kangaroos that stumbled into a hornets' nest—it keeps constantly jumping off in all directions. You don't learn to do it better each time, and don't expect to or you will be sorely disappointed. The very design of meditation makes this impossible. If anyone tells you he meditates without distractions and coming back over and over, it means that as soon as he starts he trances out or "blisses out." These are very pleasant things to do, but they have little to do with meditating.

One other aspect of this is not to have any expectations as to how a particular session will go. The fact that you have had three "good" sessions does not in any way imply that the fourth will be either good or bad. Anything real in human feelings or reactions is unpredictable. There are just too many factors (we don't even know what most of them are!) to be able to predict. Feeling in advance that a session should be particularly good, bad, or anything else, or that it should be just like a previous session, is most likely to lead to an attempt to imitate that other session and thus to make it a ritual rather than real. Anything that is authentic about our experiences always has an element of the new and unexpected in it. If we are not somewhat surprised by an experience, it is not likely to have much effect on us.

Why do our minds resist meditation so vehemently? We do not know. However, this has been reported on by all serious students of the practice from the ancient Greeks to Catholic saints like St. Theresa of Avila to Eastern wisdom seekers like Ramakrishna. Some have tried to explain it, some have not, but all noted it and its strength and all have said you simply have to keep struggling through it. In all probability you will invent some interesting ways to resist the discipline yourself. If you are smart about this, you will note when—or soon after—you do it, congratulate yourself on being so clever, wish you could use the same amount of cleverness in your daily life, and get back to your meditation program. As we discuss specific meditations, I will describe some of the more common forms of resistance to each of them. The most common overall is either falling asleep or suddenly realizing that for a period of time when you were supposed to be working you were thinking of something else entirely or just letting your mind drift.

How do you handle it when you find you are thinking of something else rather than meditating? You can call yourself stupid and weak and resolve not to think of that other subject anymore. This is a common, but certainly not a recommended reaction. Or you can say, "There, there, honey, that's because you are a human being and that's how human beings act in meditation. Come on, dear, back to work." This is the recommended way. To treat yourself like a much loved child whom you want to keep walking on the sidewalk. The child dashes off to one side to climb a lovely apple tree. You make a long arm and pull the child back to the sidewalk and smile at it. The child dashes off to the other side to smell a beautiful flower. Again you reach out and say, "That's what children do, dear, but let's get back on the sidewalk now." In other words, you demand the best of yourself, but with love, humor, gentleness. You treat yourself as you wish you were treated as a child, as you would like to be able to treat a child you love, and as we hope and pray that someday all the children in the world will be treated.

This special attitude toward yourself is one of the most important parts or aspects of meditation, and also one of the least written about or taught. In developing and using this attitude toward yourself, you provide a sort of special nourishment or "top soil" that is ideal for, and makes much easier, future growth in healthy directions. It is literally the nourishment we need to keep developing as human beings in positive ways.

Just as one form of physical exercise is best for one person and another is best for a second, so meditations also vary in their appropriateness for each person. There is no one best way to meditate just as there is no one best way to exercise and no one best diet for everyone.

You may find that a particular meditation is not right for you—that it arouses negative and anxious feelings. This is very rare with the meditations presented in this book, but it does happen occasionally. By negative feelings I do not mean boredom or "I wish I were anywhere but here." All meditation will make you feel that way at one time or another.

Once in a long while, however, a particular meditation technique will make a specific person feel anxious or depressed. If this happens, switch to an alternate meditation. (In all my experience I have never encountered the situation where both alternatives produced a negative reaction.) Do not be brave and go on in spite of the negative feelings. Heroics have no place in real personality growth. Hard and consistent work do have a central and very real place, but not heroics.

As long as I am on the subject of individual differences and some meditations being better for you than others, let me mention again that there is no single diet that is right for everyone. Find the best diet for you at this stage of your development. What is a good diet for one person is wrong for another and any nutritionist who uses the same diet for everyone is hopelessly bigoted and outdated.

I learned this and had it repeatedly reinforced when working with people with cancer. There was no one correct or best diet for all of them. For example, there is a widely publicized diet called the Macrobiotic Diet. During the years I worked in the cancer field I saw people who did very well on it. I also saw many who did very poorly on it and in whom it produced negative effects.

Certainly there are some good general rules. If, however, you use a nutritionist, find one who does not rely only on them or on a particular fad which seems attractive and well publicized at the moment. A good nutritionist should ask many questions—before prescribing a diet. He or she should ask what foods give you energy and do not cause you to "crash" afterward. What foods are addictive for you so that if you eat them you want more? Are you a "breakfast," a "lunch," or a "supper" person?

Are you a one or two or three or four or five meals a day person or a snacker? And so forth and so on. And then, in conjunction with you, the good nutritionist will work out a diet. On the one hand the ideal team consists of a medical or professional expert who knows the field and its resources. On the other hand it needs the world's outstanding authority on how you feel and your experience—you. When these two operate as a team of equals, there is a far better chance of achieving good results than with any other combination I know.

~

MEDITATION IS NOT EASY. You will find it hard work, and work that requires all your attention. Whether the particular meditation you are working with is as rigorous as Contemplation (Chapter 2) or as gentle as the Safe Harbor meditation (Chapter 4) it still requires that you follow the rules and focus your consciousness to stay with it.

There are forms of meditation which are much easier than those presented here. These are restful and pleasant and are certainly good for you. One form, for example, tells you to just lie back, allow your mind to wander as it pleases with no particular program, and every time nothing is going on, to repeat a specific phrase (mantra) to yourself. Doing this for two twenty-minute periods each day is undoubtedly beneficial. What a nice gift to give to yourself—forty minutes a day with no goals, nothing to do except to be!

By and large, however, this type of work does not lead to real change. We might make again the analogy to a gymnasium. This approach is like going to the gym and relaxing in the whirlpool, sitting in the steam room, and having a massage. Very good for you, but if you want real change in your muscular or cardiovascular system, you have to do real, sweat-producing work. You have to jog or lift weights or push a Nautilus machine or ride a stationary bicycle or something like that. The meditations in this book are of that sort. Their goal is to produce the kind of change that will enable you to take more control of your eating habits and of your life generally.

⌒

IN THE FOLLOWING chapters, I will discuss each of the four parts of the program for achieving an ideal body weight. These are:

1. Meditations to discipline the mind and to learn to cope better with problems and temptations. Chapter 2.

2. Meditations designed for the specific purpose of weight management. Chapter 3.

3. Meditations to help in the especially hard parts of your program and the times when you feel you are going to fail at it. Chapter 4.

4. Meditations and exercises to help you upgrade your life overall and to find new sources of satisfaction other than food. Chapter 7.

Read the entire book. Then, to start, choose one exercise from Chapter 2 and one from Chapter 3. The way to choose is to try each of them three or four times for fifteen minutes each. Then choose the two you are going to work with, decide on the amount of time you will work with each one every day, and commit yourself to a set period for doing this. I would suggest a period of four, five, or six weeks. Then you make a promise to yourself that you will do this no matter what happens unless an overwhelming emergency interferes. By an overwhelming emergency I mean one of the caliber that involves paramedics with an ambulance or a squad of firefighters coming to your home. Short of this kind of disaster, you are committed. At the end of the period you have selected, reevaluate. You may want to change one of the meditations you are using or the amount of time you are working each day.

If it gets too difficult and you feel—during the initial period—that you simply will not be able to continue, choose one of the exercises in Chapter 4—exercises for the hard and discouraging moments—and add this to your program. Do not substitute it for one of the other meditations you have chosen, but add it on. Choose it in the same way you did the others—experiment with all those given in the chapter, choose one, and commit yourself to it.

There will be hard times. Growth and change are never easy. You are in this work learning to take control of an area of your life that has been causing you much pain and sorrow. If it were easy, you would have done it long ago. But you can learn to be in control by taking control of your own meditation program. You will be taking charge of yourself.

A number of years ago, a group of tough, adolescent gang kids were talking to the head worker in an open drop-in center that had been established in New York's Bedford Stuyvesant area. (A place where policemen go in threes!) She mentioned meditation and the kids asked her about it. After a few minutes of explanation, she asked if they wanted her to teach them about it. They replied that they didn't want her, but the person who had taught her. She called me and I went down one morning. Two of them met me at the subway station and escorted me so that I would arrive safely at the center. There were fifteen of them and the first question they asked was about the purpose of meditation—why do it? I looked at this tough group, every one of whom knew how to handle a pusher or a parole officer and could instantly spot the faintest sign of phoniness in a middle-class, middle-aged white like me. I knew I had to reply with complete honesty. I said, "It's to help you learn to be the boss of you. To drive your own car and not let the direction or speed be chosen by your impulses of the moment or because of what others tell you, or how you feel at any moment. It's to learn to run your own show." I have never seen a group work harder and more consistently than those fifteen adolescents did that long day we worked together.

So if you are ready to commit yourself to learning how to run your own life, at least in the weight management area, turn to the next chapter and let us begin.

# ·2·

≈

# The First Meditations
# for Your Program

*O*N THIS CHAPTER you will find a number of meditations that, if practiced regularly, will help you learn to work with your own mind, will give you confidence in your ability to do this, and will generally increase your ability to cope with both internal and external problems. They will also quickly cure you of the idea that you, or anyone else for that matter, can learn to meditate expertly and well. St. Theresa of Avila once said, "The mind of an adult is like an unbroken horse. It will go in any direction except the one in which you want it to go." You will quickly find out how true this is. The important thing about this kind of work is to do it because doing it helps you accomplish your goals, not to learn to do it well. It is sort of like the experience of riding a stationary bicycle in the gymnasium. You do not expect to get anywhere, but the experience itself is good for you!

The first of these exercises will be one widely used by Eastern meditation groups. It is called Breath Counting.

In this exercise—as in all of the "inner" or nonbody-movement meditations, you start by getting comfortable. Loosen your clothing and take off your shoes if this is possible. Lean back in your armchair, stretch out on the floor, or get into whatever position is best for you. By best, I mean that position which is least likely to interrupt your work by causing cramps or discomfort.

Now focus your attention on your breathing. At each exhalation count "one," "two," "three," "four," "one," "two," and so forth. It is generally easier if you put an "and" between each count to fill up the time when you are inhaling. Do not try to change or modify the rhythm of breathing, just count your exhalations. The goal is to be as awake, alert, and aware as possible and to be doing only one thing—counting your breaths. Whenever you realize (as you frequently will) that you have drifted off from this, say, in effect, "That's what we humans do, honey. Now back to work." Then refocus your thoughts and get back to the procedure.

Your goal is to be so involved in doing this that you are not even aware you are doing it. The violinist playing a passage of music is completely focused on what he is doing. Wide awake, completely alert, at the peak of awareness, there is only the focusing on the action and the action itself in consciousness. There is no consciousness of "Now I am playing the violin." Nor is there a sense of "Now we are going to repeat the earlier theme." He is simply playing the violin and that is what he is aware of. Similarly the mechanic who is trying to adjust a carburetor. There is in her consciousness only the action and the awareness of the action. There are no "Now I am adjusting a carburetor" thoughts. There is simply total focus; what is called in the East "Bare Attention." Both the violinist and the mechanic are totally focused on what they are doing, with as few extraneous thoughts as a dog who is pointed at a rabbit. From his nose to his tail, the dog is just pointing at the rabbit—that is all. But he is doing it actively and totally.

Do not be discouraged when you find that you spend

most of your time drifting off, realizing that you have drifted off, and bringing yourself back. That is what everyone else does too. Unless they have "tranced out" or "blissed out." It is the work itself that is good for us—that builds muscles and control.

Try this for five minutes. Now.

Now think about the experience you have just had. I am sure you now know what St. Theresa meant in her comment about the mind being like an unbroken horse! Think about how your life would be if you had as little control over your body as you do over your mind. You would never get down a flight of stairs alive. One foot would go this way, the other that way!

Now set yourself for a serious tryout of this meditation. Try it for fifteen minutes. Now.

How do you feel? Ask yourself and look within for the answer. Think about it. How did it go? You have just had an experience with a "structured," "discipline" meditation. You have had an experience working with your own mind. Review the experience.

After each meditation period, try to take a few minutes—perhaps 10 or 15 percent of the total time of the meditation experience—to just "be." Do not have any agenda, any program for this time. Just remain physically quiet and allow what happens in your mind to happen. In a sense you are allowing your self to "digest" the experience. After that, ask yourself how you feel and look within to find out. Do this with all meditations as a regular practice. If the timing device you have put within easy eye range has a big sweep second hand, it will be easier to time this "no agenda" period. Many people find it very hard to allow themselves a period of time with no agenda or program. They get uncomfortable and somehow feel they should be doing something. Ask yourself if you feel this way. If you do, take the time anyway and simply observe your feelings of discomfort. If you stay with the practice and follow these directions, after a time the feelings will ease. You will have learned something about "being," something you already know about "doing." For many of us, this is a new lesson.

One technique you may discover yourself using to resist the discipline is the sudden insight into the solution of a problem you have been working on for some time. Few of us would be silly enough to go on with the meditation, letting go and possibly forgetting the suddenly realized answer to a question with which we have been concerned. On the other hand, we have made ourselves a promise to work for a specific period. The best way to deal with this is to quickly glance at the clock, then pick up a pencil and paper and write down the new insight. Take as long as you need to be sure you will not lose it. Then look at the clock again, figure out what the time will be when you finish the meditation, go back to it, and—giving it the full treatment—complete it. Thus you will have worked for as long as you promised yourself and you will still have the insight. You have your cake and have eaten it also!

THE SECOND MEDITATION in this chapter is used in a very wide variety of meditational schools, both Eastern and Western. It is called Contemplation. Of all the meditational forms, this is probably the second most common. (The one used most often is the "mantra" described in Chapter 3.) The way I will describe it and the instructions I give here come primarily from Western sources. (Most particularly from Evelyn Underhill's *Practical Mysticism,* arguably the best and clearest book on the meditational path ever written.)

First you will need an object to contemplate. I strongly advise a small seashell or a piece of a larger one, a crystal, an interesting pebble, or a semiprecious stone. In other words, a nature object that is interesting and durable. Another possibility is something like a small piece of jewelry that is not very ornate and does not have any particular emotional connotations for you.

Get yourself comfortable. Then begin to look at your object. Not to talk about it to yourself or even to use words, but simply to look. If you had a piece of velvet and wanted to know its texture you would run your hand over it and concentrate on the sensation in your palm and fingers. You would not be likely to use words but would try simply to be aware of the sensations in your hands. Similarly, if you were listening to a piece of good music well played, you would not —if you were really listening—be describing it or your activity to yourself in words. You would not be saying to yourself things such as, "Here the music is derivative of Beethoven," or "Here is where the oboe comes to the forefront." In other words, there is a difference between functioning as a listener and functioning as a music critic. To listen, you are highly aware, highly alert, and just listening.

When you find, as you are looking at the object you have chosen for contemplation, that you are using words, you smile indulgently at yourself, and say, in effect, "That's how it goes with us humans, dear," and pull yourself back to work. Shortly you will have to repeat the process. And again and again. Remember, nobody meditates well. We all just work at it.

"Caress it with your eyes," wrote Evelyn Underhill. "Regard it the way a contented cat broods on the ultimate mouse." Look. Look. Look. "I do not require of you," said St. Theresa of Avila, "any deep and serious considerations in your thinking. I require you only to look." Look at the contemplation object as you would look at the face of one you love—no words or descriptions, just a deep desire to know the face.

Try this for five minutes—now.

After the five minutes, take a minute or longer with no agenda. Remain as you are physically and let what happens in your mind happen. Now review the experience. What was it like? How do you feel now? Mentally explore yourself and see how you feel.

When you are ready, try a full fifteen minutes with this exercise. Over the next few days you will want to do this three or four times before deciding whether or not to include it in your meditation program.

Do not be surprised to find that you have a great deal of resistance to this form of meditation. In fact it would be very surprising if you did not! Dozing off is one common resistance. Another is what the Zen group calls "Makyo." These are simple hallucinations apparently produced by certain parts of the mind to fight the discipline of the exercise. You may see an aura around the meditation object. Or you may see it accordion in size, getting smaller and larger. Or feel currents running through your body. Or you may feel heavier or lighter or whatnot. An ancient Hindu manuscript written about six centuries before Christ lists fifty of these hallucinations. Then it states "But these are only the most common types!" As with other forms of resistance, the best way to handle these is to feel proud of your cleverness in finding ways of resisting the discipline, to wish you could show as much creativity in your everyday life, and to get on with your business. Every serious meditational school has warnings against taking this kind of thing seriously. Typical of these is the story of the advanced student who was studying with the Zen master Dogen. One day he went to Dogen and said, "Master, yesterday while sitting in the lotus position and meditating, I saw a great white light with the Buddha behind it!" Dogen answered him, "That's nice, if you concentrate on your breathing it will go away!"

⌒

THE THIRD EXERCISE in this chapter is also a structured discipline meditation. In this one you visualize a point of light traveling slowly around the surface of your body.

Again, start by getting comfortable. Close your eyes. Then visualize a small circle of light, perhaps a quarter to a half inch across, on the palm of your right hand. Once you have it clearly in your mind's eye, make it travel *slowly* around to the back of your hand and then up the outside of your arm. Make it do this slowly and have it cover each inch, no skipping! Then make it travel up your neck, over your right ear and the top of your head, and down the other side and the other arm. When you reach the back of your left hand, make it move around to the palm and then up the inside of your arm to the armpit. Then have it go, still slowly, down the side of your body. Midway down the chest have it travel around the chest, then down to the waist, around the waist, down to the hips and around. Then make it go down the outside of your left leg, under the arch of your foot, up the inside of the left leg to the groin, down the inside of the right leg, under the foot, up the outside of the leg and the side of the body to the right armpit, and down the inside of the right arm until it slowly reaches the palm where you started.

If you lose your concentration during the course of the journey, you do not have to go back to the beginning and start over. Just go back to the last place on the course where you were clearly visualizing the light. Start from there and go on. Do this as many times as is necessary until you finish the trip.

This meditation is less complex than it appears on first

reading. After doing it once or twice, the directions will be clearly in your mind and not confusing. For most people, the hardest part is making the light travel around the chest, waist, and hips. Hopefully, as you go on with the program, this will get to be a shorter and shorter distance!

After the first experience with this meditation, try to adjust the speed of movement of the light so that the entire trip takes somewhere around fifteen minutes. You are in control of this exercise as you want to be in control of your weight and your own life.

After you have done the meditation, take the one and a half or two full minutes with no agenda. Simply let your mind do whatever it does. Then review the experience. How was it? How do you feel now?

TRY EACH OF these three meditations three or four times. Spend about fifteen minutes on each meditation. Then choose one to work with on a regular basis, five or seven times a week. (Some people have such complex weekend schedules that it is better for them to choose five times a week, as they will not keep to the program if they plan to work on Saturday or Sunday.) Then pick the amount of time for your first work period. I suggest a six-week period although you may prefer four or five, or seven or eight. Whatever you pick, you are now committed. You have made a promise to yourself and if you are going to learn to treat yourself with respect and with love, you will keep it.

Before you get started on this program, however, you will need to pick an exercise from Chapter 3. When you are ready, go to this new chapter and follow the instructions for choosing a meditation.

# ·3·

# Specific Meditations
# for Weight Control

*I*N THIS CHAPTER there will be described two meditations specifically designed to help you deal with the problem of moving toward a healthy body weight. Healthy for you as an individual, not healthy according to arbitrary standards set by the fashion of the moment or by the advertising agencies. To do this, your diet must be determined primarily by the needs of your body, not by your eating habits, your whims, or your emotional needs. As you read and explore the meditations described in this chapter, you will understand their relationship to this change.

Read the instructions for each meditation. Try each one three or four times. Then choose one for your program for the next four to eight weeks—the period you have decided to work before reevaluating the situation and deciding either to continue with the program you have or else to modify it.

In addition to the two meditations from which you will choose one for your program, there are two others, to be done before eating or at mealtimes. These should be a part of the work for everyone who is using this book to achieve a healthy body weight.

⌒

The first of the meditations specifically concerned with dieting is generally called the Thousand Petal Lotus technique. It is widely used, particularly in Eastern meditational schools. In its original form, it was designed to help the meditator realize that everything in the universe is connected to everything else and that:

> All things, by immortal power,
> Near and far, hiddenly,
> To each other linked are,
> That thou cannot stir a flower
> Without troubling of a star.

This was its original purpose, but it has also been adapted to a number of special problems, as we are adapting it here to the problem of weight control. It is a meditation of "the inner way" in which we meditate on the activity of our own consciousness rather than on an object (as a seashell) or an activity (as our own breathing) outside of our consciousness.

We begin by choosing one word as the "center" of the lotus. Pick a word such as "hungry," "diet," "thin," "fat," or your favorite "binge" food. (Mine are Mallomars, but choose your own.) Then get comfortable, "regard" the word, and simply wait. Sooner or later you will have an association to the word. Suppose you have chosen the word hungry and your first association is "full." You now have three things— the word hungry, the word full, and the connection between them. Do you understand the connection or not? In this case you do. You know quickly what the relationship is between these two words and why you made the association. You then go back to "hungry," regard it, and wait for the next association. Suppose this next one is "starving." Again, you look at the three things for five or six seconds. And again you understand the connection. You go back again to "hungry," and wait, just as you did before. Suppose the next association is "roof." You look at the three for the five or six seconds and this time you do not understand the connection. You still go back to "hungry" and wait. And so on for the full time you allotted in advance to this meditation. You respond the same way—regarding the two words and their connection for five or six seconds and then going back to the center word and waiting—whether or not you understand the connection.

This is not free association in which you just go from one association to the next. You always go back to the word you have chosen for the center. Nor do you try to "understand" anything except whether or not you make sense of the connection between the center and the association. No matter how juicy and tempting the lead, whether or not it seems to indicate deep insights into the workings of your unconscious, just stay with the discipline. Insights are to be tasted and possibly explored *after* the meditation, not during it. When you violate this rule, and you will, you will find that, as a resistance technique, all sorts of fascinating insights are suggested by the associations, but that they do not pan out. They turn out to be fluff with no substance. Real insights will appear from this meditation if you follow it vigorously, but they will appear after you have finished a good number of sessions, not during them (and particularly not during or after the first few sessions).

This is the most frequent form of resistance to appear with this meditation—the strong feeling that if you abandon the discipline and follow up an idea that has come up from the associations, or go on with a free association technique, you will learn something fascinating about yourself, about others, or about the workings of the universe. These feelings are red herrings and will successfully lead you away from the meditation and any value you can get out of it until you learn successfully to resist them. However, practically no one learns this except through experience. So, do your best not to violate the discipline in this way, smile ruefully at yourself when you find you have done so and joined the club, and get back to work.

THE SECOND MEDITATION in this section was originally designed to help individuals to deal with certain kinds of pain. The general name for this approach is the Blue Water technique.

In this meditation, you first get comfortable and then ask yourself, "In what part of my body do I feel hunger?" Seek within your body; let your consciousness rove all through it. Where is your hunger located? It may be in the stomach area or anywhere else. Take your time locating the source of your feeling of hunger. Explore your whole body. You will quickly find that if you are relaxed and comfortable you can aim your consciousness into any area of your body and ask, "Is this where I feel hunger?"

When you have located the area in which you feel hunger, explore its dimensions carefully. What shape is this area? How long, wide, deep is it? Visualize it as a shape with sides there, ends there, a bottom and top there.

Now visualize, imagine, this shape filling up with blue water. Never mind where it comes from. In your mind, let the water slowly fill up the space. Then imagine the water slowly draining out. Let it drain out through the walls of the space you have defined. Visualize it draining out through your skin, through the floor, and then being completely

gone, leaving never a trace, a spot, or stain of wetness behind. Then have the space fill up again with the blue water
and repeat the process. And do it once more.

The first time you do this exercise it may take some time
—perhaps up to an hour as you search first to define the area
in which you feel hunger. After that, pace yourself so that
you can repeat the filling and draining of the space two or
three times in fifteen minutes. If you can do it more rapidly
than this, you are going too fast. Slow it down.

The most common resistance to this meditation is to put
it "on automatic." It goes on—usually faster and faster—
while your mind goes in other directions and you think of
other things. Do it with as total concentration as you can and
keep control of the pace.

After the exercise, take some "no agenda, no program"
time. Then ask yourself how you feel, and look within for the
answer.

☜

IN ADDITION TO the meditation you have chosen for your
weight program, there is another that everyone should do. (If
you find it very distasteful or unpleasant, as a very few people do, then skip it. Otherwise include it.) This is not done
during your meditation periods, but at mealtimes. Try to do
it for one meal every day. If this is too difficult because of the
way your life is organized, then do it once, for one meal,
every other day.

This meditation is a very old one used in both Eastern
and Western meditation schools. It is a form of Contemplation as described in Chapter 2. However, instead of contem-
plating (one-pointing) an object, we do it with the food we
are eating.

Eat the meal in silence and preferably alone. (Or with

someone else who is also doing the exercise.) First the food is brought to the table and you sit down to it. During eating, however, instead of letting your mind roam free or talking or reading or watching TV, or whatever you usually do, focus your consciousness as completely as possible on the sensations you feel in your mouth.

As you eat, try to be as aware as possible of what is going on in your mouth. What are you feeling, what are you tasting?

Do not worry about using words or not to describe what is going on as you eat. Just try to focus all your attention on what is going on in your mouth and what sensations you perceive. I can assure you that if you do this for a full meal you will find surprises.

The most common form of resistance to this meditation is to forget to do it at all or to keep putting it off to the next meal as this one is too inconvenient. Be warned that you will probably find yourself doing this and will probably realize suddenly that to all intents this meditation has been dropped from your program. When you realize this has happened, smile at yourself and start doing it again. It is an important part of the total program.

⌒

THE MEDITATIONS IN the second chapter—Breath Counting, Contemplation, the Circle of Light exercise—are, among other things, "centering meditations." This means that they tend to integrate you into a being who is doing one thing at a time. When we move in this direction we operate more efficiently and with less stress than we do following our usual patterns, in which we are often much more fractured. It would be fair to say that during a centering meditation, no matter how distracted we feel, the work itself brings us closer to our real needs and we function more from them than from our habits and our neurotic needs. This carries over for a period after the meditation is finished and also has a cumulative effect when we follow a regular meditation program. It is, of course, not a panacea that will solve all problems, but then we have never discovered such a thing in all the long aeons during which we human beings have looked and searched.

For this reason, it would be very helpful to your program if before each meal you chose one of the centering meditations—probably but not necessarily the one you included in your regular sessions—and did it for five minutes. This may not always be possible, but if you do it whenever you can, it will be a real help in your movement toward a healthy body weight.

One other time to do this is when you are hungry between meals, feel that you need "a little something," and that the need is strong enough that you are going to satisfy it. Delay going to the refrigerator for five minutes and work hard for this period at the centering meditation. Then, after a "no agenda" minute, ask yourself how you feel. This procedure can give you much more control over your food intake than you have had previously.

THE FOLLOWING MEDITATION is in addition to the others you have chosen, including the centering meditation just discussed. It is to be done once a day for the first two weeks of your program. Thereafter it is to be done whenever you are tempted to break your diet or to stretch it with that extra bit of bread or dessert or a between-meal snack.

Visualize an old-fashioned balance scale hanging from the ceiling directly in front of you. From each arm there hangs a bowl. There is a needle in the center with a dial behind it. The needle points directly up.

Since food is necessary to live and to be healthy, the left side of the scale facing you is white and at the bottom of the dial is the word LIFE. Since overeating is a poison to the body and poison eventually kills you, the right side of the dial is black; at the bottom is written DEATH.

Visualize the scale and the dial. When you have it fairly clear in your imagination, ask yourself in which bowl this particular bite or piece of food will go. Which way will the needle swing when and if you eat it? Get that clear in your mind. Then decide what you will do now about this particular bit of food.

Do this once a day for practice. Choose the special bit of food you are doing it with at random during the day. Do this for two weeks so that the meditation is clear to you and you know how to use it. Then, when you are about to break your diet or really wreck it with a full-scale binge, you use it. The previous practice will make it easier to do and more effective. As a meditation, it puts the food into realistic perspective. When you use it, you will be surprised how often you find you do not need, or even want, that extra slice of bread.

THERE IS A second meditational path that is possible with the material found in this book. A number of people have followed it with good success.

Sometimes in using the meditations described here, a person finds that one of them is exactly right; it fills the bill completely. Then, after following the four- to six-week program that they have promised themselves, they switch to this one and do it as a total program.

One woman was one-pointing her supper at a student center. She found the exercise exhilarating. Suddenly she was totally involved in the process of sensing what was going on in her mouth, the taste—the texture of the food, the feelings of her mouth, and so forth. The dessert served at the end of the meal was chocolate mousse, her absolute and all-her-life favorite food. She had never left a dish of it unfinished or dreamed of doing so. It seemed to her that she enjoyed the taste of it this time more than she ever had before. When she was halfway through the mousse, she realized that she had had enough. She was no longer hungry and it seemed natural to her to stop eating. She stayed with the one-pointing, doing it at least one meal a day and often two. Her pattern of bulimia seemed to clear up completely in the next several weeks and has not returned in the dozen or so years since.

As a second illustration of this, a man in his late sixties had been twenty-five to forty pounds overweight for more than twenty years. Psychotherapy had solved many problems in his life and raised his general level of functioning and his level of enjoyment. However, it had not helped his weight problem. Although he had lost weight during a stay in a yoga camp and at the Pritikin Center, it had soon returned. While getting into a meditation program, he tried the Balance Scale technique and suddenly felt strongly that this was the meditation for him. Sometimes when he was faced with food, it appeared to happen almost automatically. Whenever he thought of eating a particular food, he would imagine the balance scale in front of him with the needle pointing up. He would know if the food he was looking at would tip the needle into the white or into the black half of the dial. If it was the latter, he would lose all interest in eating it—his hunger would seem to disappear.

After finishing the five-week program he had set up for himself, he went on with only the Balance Scale meditation, making sure that he did it for at least one meal a day and usually two, and whenever he was tempted to snack in between. Over the next few months he lost the extra weight he had been carrying and felt far better than he had in years.

The kind of thing illustrated by the experiences of these two people does not happen too often, but it does happen. If you find yourself fitting this pattern—go for it! But be sure to finish the program you have promised yourself first. That way, you won't be using a single meditation as a resistance to the discipline. If you are not careful to do this, you are likely to find that the special meditation that seemed to fit you so well now no longer does, that it has become very difficult to do and no longer has any effect on you, which means that your whole program has been abandoned. You will have to start all over again. Moreover, you will have broken a promise to yourself and that is not a helpful thing for your future growth.

HARVEY WAS FORTY-SIX years old, with chocolate brown skin. He was five feet ten and 270 pounds. He had worked in construction all his life and recently had been told that unless he lost a good deal of weight he would be laid off. The engineer in charge said that it was just too dangerous for him to be working on ladders and scaffolds and the company could not afford the risk. The union shop steward had looked into the matter and told Harvey that the union could do nothing in this case except make sure he got his severance pay.

He was a very bright and able man who had found his first job in the construction field shortly after high school graduation. Except for a stint in the Army, where he was a tech sergeant in the Combat Engineers, he had worked steadily ever since. He was married with two children, both boys, one twelve and the other fourteen years old. Evenings he generally spent sitting around at home watching television, drinking a few beers with friends either at one of their houses, in his own home, or at a local bar. On his summer vacations the whole family went to the seashore. Two or three times a year he would go for a day's fishing on Long Island Sound with several friends.

His weight had slowly and steadily increased over the past ten years. He was depressed and felt that there was nothing he could do about it. He had tried various diets, but none seemed meaningful or real to him and he abandoned them all fairly early in their course. His union had suggested psychotherapy and had funds to pay most of the cost, but after one session he decided against it. He gave two reasons. First that the therapist "didn't know diddley-squat about anything" and second—"I don't want to look at all that garbage." He tried one meeting of Weight Watchers and felt completely alien and out of place. When meditation was suggested, he was quite resistant to the idea until I challenged him to do five minutes of Breath Counting and told him that if he could do it, I'd "get off his back"! He tried and found that his mind would not stay on the task. He grinned when I told him that he had about as much control over his mind as he did over his weight. Since his reponse was so positive, I went on and told him that since his mind controlled what he did and how he felt, maybe he had better start working to get some control over it if he wanted to be able to deal with the weight problem. He thought about this for a while, asked a few questions, and then smiled and said, "Okay, whitey, let's give her a try."

He chose the Breath Counting and Blue Water meditations and said he would work fifteen minutes on each one, five days a week and would set it up for six weeks. He said that it was very difficult for him to one-point a meal as breakfast was a madhouse what with getting the kids off to school and him to work, lunch was with a group of the men he worked with, and supper was the only time he and the family ever had to be together and talk. He discussed the problem with his wife, who was anxious that he lose weight. She said that every other day she would get up a few minutes earlier and bring him his breakfast on a tray in the bedroom where he could eat it alone while he did the one-pointing exercise. She also began packing more dietetic lunches for him.

He showed a sort of grim tenacity in working with the meditations. The hardest part for him was to learn not to be aggressively critical of himself when his mind wandered away from the instructions. He had a tendency to savage himself each time this happened. No matter what he tried, at first, he wound up angry at himself for not being able to "do it right." We talked a good deal about this, and eventually he began to change and to see it as a game he was teaching one of his children when they were very young—a very difficult game with complex rules. He was learning to treat himself as he wished he had been treated as a child and as he wished to treat the children he loved: firmly and demanding the best, but with love, humor, and an understanding of human weaknesses. This, of course, is the best way we know to provide the necessary terrain for future growth and change in healthy directions.

From time to time he would get terribly angry and discouraged, go off his diet and binge for a few days. These periods seemed to be almost irrelevant to anything that was happening around him. The incidents that set them off were apparently pretty trivial and we both had the impression that he was responding more to things inside him than to outside events. I suggested that since this appeared to be so, it might be wise for him to move into the next phase, "going on from there," earlier than usual. How did he feel about the general course of his life? What, for example, about his job?

He said his job was "okay." "Paid pretty good" but was "boring, the same thing over and over year after year." What kind of work would he like to do if he had free choice? We talked about this and he did the exercises in Chapter 7 to help him clarify his goals. For the first time he became quite shy. He kept talking about helping people find the right place to go out from and to be from. I couldn't make head or tail of all this. Finally he came out with it. He would like to work as a real estate agent. He had seen agents come around with clients as a house he was working on was nearly finished and for a long time had wished he could be one of them. He looked very surprised when I asked him why he didn't go for it. After some thinking about the answer to this question, he began to attend some night school classes. My impression was that the meditation and his sticking with it had given him a confidence in his ability to do new tasks that he had never had before, and that this was one of the main factors that made the new growth and activity possible.

He enjoyed the classes. His children kidded him unmercifully, asking, "Has Pop done his homework yet?" and so forth, but they were clearly proud of him. They told all their schoolmates, and soon it was all over the neighborhood. When people he knew started coming to him with questions about moving or dealing with their landlords, he felt wonderful.

He stayed with the meditation program, but changed the Blue Water to the Thousand Petal Lotus meditation and stayed with that, using the word "food" as the center for a five-week period, then shifting to "healthy." He found that he was losing weight at a slow but steady rate and that he had no difficulty with his diet. With his friends at night (although there are far fewer of these evenings now due to his classes and homework) he sticks to two or three "light" beers. He found the Balance Scale meditation very helpful on these evenings.

I talked with his wife. She understood and approved of what Harvey was doing, but seemed a little surprised when I asked her what she would do, how she would grow when it became her turn. I told her that if two people were close and one changed in a positive direction, it was important for the other to do the same. Otherwise there was a real possibility that they would grow apart. She thought about this and presently started going to the church two evenings or so a week and helping the man who did the church bookkeeping. She started as a sort of "gofer" and in a year was doing most of the actual work. She enjoys this and said that on the job was the best way for her to learn as she had never done very well at school. Her goal is to do the accounting and bookkeeping for a small business in the neighborhood as a part-time profession.

Harvey is now working as a real estate agent in a small agency two or three days a week. He is still studying for his license. He enjoys this work very much and is apparently quite good at it. He and his wife had to dip into their savings as the money he now earns is less than he received in full-time construction work, but they expect to get back to where they had been financially in the near future. He gets plenty of exercise in the construction work he does the other three days a week. His weight is now one hundred and ninety, and he feels fine. He and his wife say that their life is good and busy and they feel they are on a good track.

Harvey was unusual in that he and I saw each other frequently during the course of his program. People differ in the amount of personal help and contact they need when using the meditational route. Some can do it by themselves, following a book like this one, which is written partially for that purpose. Others need more or less personal interaction with a specialist.

## ·4·

### ⌒

# When the Pressures Get Too Heavy:
# Meditations for
# Especially Difficult Times

*Y*OU NOW HAVE an individual
meditation program to help you move toward a healthy body
weight. This is probably something you have wanted for a
long time and have made a number of attempts to achieve.
You have chosen a basic centering exercise (Breath Counting,
Contemplation, or the Circle of Light), and one specific meditation oriented to the problem of weight control (the Thousand Petal Lotus or the Where Am I Hungry? meditation).
You are one-pointing your food for one meal a day or for one
meal every other day. For the first two weeks you are also
using the Balance Scale meditation. In addition, at those special moments when you find yourself going for (as Pooh
would have put it) "a little smackeral of something" you are
now delaying opening the refrigerator door for five minutes
while you do a quick and hard centering meditation.

This is, indeed, a good basic program. However, you also
need to be prepared for those special times when stress has
built up to the degree that you know you are going to break
your diet and reach for the comfort of extra and biologically
unneeded food in the next few minutes—if there is one more
telephone call informing you that all your carefully and labo-

riously worked-out plans have been canceled, one more thing in your immediate environment that is going to stop functioning, or one more person needing or asking for something from you. And, further, you know, based on the record of all your experience, that one or more of these things is going to happen. How do you handle this kind of special stress, which is making you feel as if you have been starving for a week and which is clearly going to make you go on automatic pilot and start eating for comfort and emotional survival, as you have done so often in the past? A meditation program for a healthy body weight is a fine idea no doubt, but can it handle the special times when stress builds so high that you know you are shortly going to use that old technique of yours—eating to relieve the pressure? A long habit of eating food you do not biologically need in difficult times is bound to wreak havoc with many programs. To say nothing of the problems it will create in your long-term weight situation unless you get the habit under control. In this chapter, I will describe some special meditations for use in these times. These are to be added to your usual program, not substituted for them. When the going gets really rough, try each of these three or four times. Then pick one to add to your program.

It may be most helpful if you *assume* there will be extra-difficult times and prepare in advance. This means taking the time early in your program to carefully read this chapter, try out each of the meditations a few times, and, in this way, get a real sense of them. Then, when you hit a rough period, you will be in a better position to make a choice. And you are almost certain to hit such rough periods. Modern life (perhaps all life) is complex and unpredictable. The best laid plans of mice and men often fail at the last moment. Life is often difficult, uncertain, and painful.

The first meditation for use in difficult times is called the

Safe Harbor meditation. It is a development of a technique originally described by the spiritual development arm of the Eastern Orthodox Church in about the seventh century A.D. There, in the Syrian-Jordanian deserts, this group (known as the Hesychiast School), calling their way of working the Way of Sweet Repose, devised this approach. They named it the Meditation on the Light in the Center of the Flame.

Get yourself physically at ease in whatever position you use for meditation. Visualize yourself comfortably located in a warm and pleasant formless area, a place without any shapes in it, with no sharp visual images, no loud sounds or strong smells. Perhaps you are sitting relaxed in a gentle gray fog or in a twilight dimness. Without using your muscles and with no effort, you are able to move your body at will in both time and space. Wait and "put out your antennae," "listen" for a faint signal. It may be faint music or a sense of light coming from one "direction." It may be a humming, or a feeling of pleasant tension in one "direction," or any other faint but real sort of signal. It is from a time and place, a moment in your past where and when, for a period, you were completely fulfilled. Where if you had been asked, you would have added or subtracted or changed nothing. Where you could have said to the moment, "Stop there, you are so beautiful." This experience in your past is sending out a faint signal through the formless place where you are. Let yourself become aware of the signal and gently will yourself to move, to drift, in the "direction" in time and place from which it is coming.

As you move yourself through the formless area toward the source of the signal, you find that moment in your past life waiting for you. It is there as if it were happening now. Enter the moment, reexperience it to the fullest. Live it again. Sense how you felt there. Stay with it as long as you need to —as long as it feels "right." Then, as you leave the full experience, remembering it with all your being, ask yourself about it. During that period, how were you relating to yourself, to others, to the world as a whole? Was the universe friendly as you were experiencing it? How were you "balanced" inside yourself? How much were you relating to the present moment, to the past, to the future?

This moment, this experience, fulfilled a part of you. However, as Plato pointed out so long ago, we each have many parts. Return in your inner life to the formless place. Bring with you the experience you have just remembered and felt and lived again. Wait for the first signs of another signal. Be patient if it does not come immediately. It will come. Again follow it to its source, moving yourself mentally and without effort in the direction it comes from. It will soon lead you to another experience in your past where another part of you was so fulfilled that during the period it was going on, you would have changed nothing. Enter this second experience, relive it, have and feel it again to the fullest as you did with the first. Stay as long as you need or wish to. Then as you leave, ask yourself about it as you did before. What part of you did this one fulfill? How, when you were in it, did you relate to yourself, to others, and to the world as a whole?

Reexperiencing one or two of these special moments should take you up to half an hour or so. But it may legitimately take longer—you may do only one in a half-hour or so. Or you may not finish with the first and need to go back to it in the next one or several sessions. Any faster and you are rushing the meditation and not letting yourself experience it to the full. After the meditation, just let yourself "be" where you are—let your mind and feelings do as they do—impose no plans or agenda for at least three to five minutes. (Decide before the meditation how long this period will be.) Then ask yourself how you feel now.

When you repeat this procedure at another time—preferably the next day—try not to have any expectations as to what the meditation will be like. It may or may not be similar to the previous one or ones. The experience or experiences you "drift" yourself toward and reenter may or may not be the same ones. The feelings during and after may be similar or dissimilar.

If you decide to include this meditation in your program, do it for a serious amount of time—for three, four, five, or six weeks, depending on what period you choose when you begin the program as a whole. You would not expect any real results from one or two gymnasium workouts with a weight machine. It is only over a serious amount of time that the results show. The same is true of meditating. Whether we are talking about physical, mental, emotional, or spiritual areas (or all or some of them at once), we humans have found no way to speed up the process of real growth and development. Do not expect this—or any other meditation—to be a "rapid method." We have never found one yet. Anyone who tells you about one (or tries to sell you one) is either a fool or a liar.

If done consistently over a serious amount of time, this Meditation on the Light in the Center of the Flame tends to lead to feelings of serenity and of being at home with yourself, with others, and in the universe generally. It also tends to provide a "safe harbor," a way of being that you can go to in times of stress, pressure, or pain. It leads to the comprehension of a way of being that is so "right" for you as an individual that it brings inner and outer harmony with it. Each of the special experiences we relive in this exercise reflects one part of the special style and way of being in the world that is naturally ours—one part of the total Safe Harbor. Together they form a way of being that helps bring us to our unique inner strength and peace—to our serenity.

It is a wonderful inner "place" to go to in moments of psychological distress and at those times when you feel you are about to be overwhelmed by the pressure of events. You might use it, go to it, in a short rest period during a long and frustrating day, the evening before you are going to have surgery, sitting in a dentist's chair, or when you feel life is simply too much and you are going to *have* to binge on food.

A SECOND MEDITATION we can use in those difficult moments when the pressure of outside events interacts with our habitual patterns of eating for emotional needs (and not in relation to our biological needs) and threatens to wreck our program for achieving our best body weight, is called a mantra. Of all the meditational forms, this is the most widely used the world over.

In a mantra, you choose a verbal phrase and repeat it over and over again. You are attempting to be as alert, as aware, as awake as possible and simply to be conscious of one thing—the phrase you are repeating. Each time you notice that your attention has wandered away to something else, you smile at yourself, say to yourself (in effect), "That's how we humans are, dear," and bring yourself back to the mantra.

It is best if you repeat the phrase aloud. Use a quiet voice, but one that is more than a whisper, a voice that involves your vocal cords. In many situations, of course, this is not possible due to the presence of others who would react and distract you and spoil your concentration. Under these conditions, simply say the mantra silently to yourself. This is not chanting or singing. It is speaking a phrase over and over, vocally or subvocally, and trying to "hear" its meaning.

You repeat the mantra steadily for the time you allotted

to the meditation before you began. I suggest that you choose a fifteen- or twenty-minute period.

You will have—in all probability—to get through a good deal of resistance in the first few sessions. This will be likely to include finding other—and often humorous—meanings in the phrase, discovering that it seems to you to be completely meaningless, finding that the whole procedure appears to be the silliest and possibly most stupid thing in which you have ever been involved, and similar developments. Deal with these as you deal with the other resistances that have appeared as you worked with your meditational program— congratulate yourself on the creativity you have shown by being so ingenious in inventing and using resistance methods, wish you could have as much creativity and ingenuity in your everyday life, and get on with your program!

You may do this meditation while walking—on a route which you know well and on which you will not be interrupted or have to cross any street with traffic. (This last so you will not have to break your concentration in order to survive.) A path used for running or jogging is often adequate. Or you can do this meditation while sitting or lying down comfortably. Whatever position you use, make sure to keep your spine straight enough so that your chest is not constricted.

Choose a phrase and then stay with it. No changing in the middle. Once you select a phrase you are stuck with it for the fifteen- or twenty-minute period you have chosen for the three or four or five weeks on which you have decided. You have made a promise to yourself. And part of any serious meditational program is learning how to keep promises to yourself.

Choose a phrase that makes sense in terms of the situation. For example, in this program you are trying to take control of your own life, to be in charge of your actions and your destiny. Choose a phrase relevant to this.

Widely used mantras in other times and places have included "God is good," "All is one," *"Kyrie Eleison* (Lord, have mercy)," "I have heard no bad news," "O God, come to my aid" *(Deus in adiutorium meum intende),* the Eastern "A U M" (a four-syllable phrase—the A, the U, the M, and the silence!), and others. These were relevant to the problems people were working on there and then. Choose one that is relevant to you here and now:

"I am in charge of my body"

"I will run my own life"

"I will cherish and protect my body"

"I am the boss of me"

"I will take as good care of my body as I do of my (cat, car, child—*choose one or substitute your own)*

"I will not damage myself"

"I will act as if I truly loved me"

"I will protect my body as I would a loved child"

Or design your own

THE LAST EXERCISE in this chapter—devoted to those times when the stress of life is too great and you are about to (or have just) abandoned your plans to work toward a healthy body weight—is of a type different from the others we have discussed so far. It involves another meaning of the term "meditation."

In this definition of meditation you read or follow a paragraph or passage of writing that is relevant to solving the problem with which you are involved. You do this slowly and with as much focus as you can bring to bear. You try to read and to *hear* at the same time; to read the words and hear the meaning. You let the words and their meaning resonate through you. You pay the fullest attention you can to the passage.

When you come to it, read the passage at the end of this section. It will be in darker typescript. If it is at all possible in your situation, read it aloud. If this is not possible, read it "subvocally"—that is, reading it as if you were reading it aloud, moving your mouth and lips, but not activating the air stream of your voice or your vocal chords. In effect, you are reading it aloud but not making a sound!

Take your time. After you have read it *slowly,* with as much intent to hear it as possible, take a few minutes (having decided in advance how long this will be—I suggest three or four minutes), with no agenda or plans. Just be physically comfortable and let what happens in your mind and feelings happen. Then repeat the entire procedure.

Do this a third time. Then, after the "no plans or agenda" period ask yourself how you feel at this moment. Look and feel within for the answer. Stay with the answer for a minute or two.

If you choose this meditation, include it as an addition to your regular program. Promise yourself that you will do it each day when you do the rest of your program for the specific number you have chosen at the start. (I suggest three or four or five.) Carry out this promise.

As with the other meditations in this book, this one seems far simpler than it is. As you go on with it, you will find yourself hearing and responding to different levels and different meanings in the words and sentences. Over time, it can be very effective.

> My body and I are one. How I treat my body is how I treat myself. What I do to my body shows how I feel about myself, my being, my hopes, my fate.
>
> I may not be able at this time to change my feelings about the kind of person I am and what kind of life I truly deserve and truly desire for me.
>
> But I can *act* as if I cared deeply and lovingly for me. I can take charge and treat my body as if I cherished and loved and had high hopes for myself. I can control my actions.
>
> I cannot decide what my feelings, wishes, desires are or will be. But I can decide how I respond and will respond to them. I am in full charge of my muscles and my actions. I can *decide* how much and what I eat and how much and how I exercise. I can decide how I will treat myself. I am in control of my actions.
>
> I know that the best way to develop good feelings about myself is to act as if I were worth caring for and cherishing. But whatever my feelings and desires are or may be, I am in charge of how I *act* toward myself. I have the power to treat myself with love.

There was once a great French philosopher named Pascal. He was a deeply serious man who is not known ever to have said a superficial thing in his life. (He invented conic geometry at the age of sixteen, which I personally find rather frightening!) He lived in an age when the great questions with which people were concerned involved their faith in the existence and goodness of God. Once he was asked, "What should a person do if he loses his faith?" He replied, "Act as if you have faith and faith will come." This is a deeper response than appears at first glance and has much truth in it.

Today we have other basic questions and the great questions of Pascal's age do not appear as crucial or meaningful to most of us. Further, we have a great deal of information he did not have and could not have had in the seventeenth century. We have, for example, learned much about the complex and dynamic qualities of the mind. But his basic insight remains valid. Our actions have a strong effect on how we feel about the world we live in, about others, and about ourselves. If we treat ourselves as if we are worth cherishing, we are very much more likely to develop strong feelings that we *are* worth cherishing. The converse of this is also true.

FOR MANY PEOPLE, the following meditation is a useful "emergency" procedure. When external and internal pressures are threatening to be too much for your weight program, try it. Do it every day for a week in addition to your regular meditation work. Then decide whether or not to continue it for a longer period. If you decide to continue, pick a definite time period during which you will do it. Then follow through. If you decide that a week is enough, you may decide to go back to it when (not if) the pressures build up again.

Get yourself physically comfortable. Do a few minutes' "centering" with one of the meditations from Chapter 2. (Breath Counting, Contemplation, or the Circle of Light). Imagine that inside your mind is a white movie screen. Visualize it. Then imagine that on this screen in a few minutes there is going to be shown a film of what your life will be like three months from now if you take control of it and yourself. Be realistic—we are not talking about your winning the lottery or moving to Camelot! The scene on the screen will be you as you would be at the healthy body weight you will achieve if you stay with the program. If you stay in control of yourself and your actions. Similarly you would have taken as much control of other aspects of your life as reality permits and upgraded them and shaped them nearer to your own heart's desire. Picture yourself after these conditions have been fulfilled. Wait for the screen to come to life. It may take time. Relax to wait. (The Buddhists say that the definition of "grace" is "patience"!) Wait and be gentle with yourself. Stay with the picture when it appears. Let it develop for fifteen minutes. On the following day repeat the process. Stay with the same scenario and develop the details or else go on with the picture to other areas and times of the day as things would be if you stayed in control of your actions and increased the areas in which you had control. After a week, decide whether or not to continue.

A form of this meditation is used by many outstanding sports figures. They picture in advance how the physical action they are about to take would be if it were done perfectly. This appears to help them perform the action as they wish to. A pole vaulter thus might visualize himself running down the approach path, placing the end of his pole correctly, lifting himself, and positioning himself perfectly over the bar. When the visualization is clear in the mind, it becomes more likely that the whole person will follow it correctly. In the same way, when we visualize exactly what we want to attain from our dieting and exercise program, it becomes more likely that we will be able to move in that direction and reach our goals.

~

THERE IS ANOTHER thing you can do to prepare for those especially hard moments that threaten you with an acute case of loss of purpose and goal. This is to sit down with yourself in advance and write out a list of things you can give yourself instead of food. As with many exercises, this one only works if it is written on paper and not just done in your mind. (For some of you who have come further into this century than I, it may be equally useful to use your computer. Intellectually I accept that this is so, even though I do not understand it emotionally!)

I learned about this method of preparation from a lovely lady who lived very close to me. One day I noticed a beautiful rosebush in her front yard. I told her my reaction to it and asked her what kind of a rose it was. She laughed and said, "I don't know what name a gardener would give it, but to me it's my ice cream rose." She went on to explain that she had been trying to diet, when one day everything seemed to go wrong. From a long planned vacation being suddenly canceled to discovering a leak in the roof that was going to cost a fortune to fix, all the stars seemed in the wrong places! She said, "It was one of those days I call 'broken shoelace days.' When you put on your shoes a shoelace breaks and you have no substitute. Then the handle comes off the coffeepot just as you are lifting it and hot coffee pours all over your new dress. Then the day goes downhill from there." She went on to say that she had gone downtown to try to straighten out a few things and put a deep scratch in the fender of her new car while trying to park it. She felt that enough was enough and she absolutely *needed* a chocolate soda to survive the next hour. On the way to the restaurant she had chosen for this, she passed a florist who had just put some rosebushes out on the sidewalk. She suddenly stopped and asked herself which would really be more comforting—the ice cream soda or a new rosebush. And then she bought what she now called her "ice cream rose."

For this exercise write out a list of things that would be

more comforting to *you* than food. Take your time and spend some thought on this. Be realistic. A voyage around the world on the *QE2* might fill the bill, but is unfortunately not in the picture for most of us. Make a list of different "ice cream roses" for yourself.

Then, whenever you feel that you are about to binge—or start starving yourself—go to the list. Look it over and ask what you could give yourself at this time that would provide you with more pleasure for a longer time than food. Then act on the answer to this question.

This exercise is part of the overall program you have embarked on. With it, you are training yourself so that when under stress you do not have to respond neurotically in the area of food, but respond instead by upgrading your life and giving yourself something much closer to what you really need. You are "comforting" yourself in the healthiest way and in a way that will increase your enjoyment of life and your self-respect rather than lessening them. In effect, this exercise is a microcosm of the entire program.

I have written in earlier chapters of the attitude it is necessary to take toward yourself while you are meditating, attempting to keep your mind highly alert, but just doing one thing at a time: that you treat yourself lovingly, firmly, gently, demanding the best but with humor and caring. This is an absolutely essential part of meditation. It is also essential if you wish to get the best out of working toward a healthy body weight. In both meditation and this work, it is best if you are very firm with yourself about one thing and make it as easy as you can for yourself about all others. In meditation, the "one thing" is following the specific instructions of the particular meditational form: for everything else, you make it as easy on yourself as possible. If you have an itch, scratch it and get back to work. If you feel cramped, stretch, rearrange your body, and get back to work. The critical thing here is to treat yourself as well as possible within the limits of the instructions.

In the overall work toward a healthy body weight, the same general concept applies. The basic factor is that you stay with and follow the instructions in your diet and exercise package—in this case the program you have set out for yourself. The rules you have set up for this package you follow as rigorously as you possibly can. You do your best not to deviate, skip, skimp, say "I'll do more tomorrow," or any other variations. But in all other respects, you treat yourself as well as you can. *Pamper yourself*, be good to yourself, buy your "ice cream rose" substitutes.

In the next chapter, I will discuss this in terms of how to maintain your newly achieved weight, but here it is important to talk about making the whole process more likely to succeed. The probability of this can be greatly increased if you generally act toward yourself as if you were really worth taking care of. You do this by being aware of yourself as a whole person and treating that person well. Be very strict in terms of calories and exercise. Be generous toward yourself in other ways.

⇒

SINCE THE EARLY 1950s, the United States has been on a dieting spree. You cannot move in this country without another diet staring you in the face. Look in at your local magazine store. No matter what day or month you do this, there will be half a dozen diets making wild claims staring you in the face.

The *New York Times* best-seller list almost invariably includes at least one diet book. (Although this is not a diet book in the usual sense of the Only Eat Strawberries and Maltose diets, I certainly hope it will replace one of them and make the list!)

Clearly these do not work. If they did, then all the people who read these magazines would long since have solved their problems and the latest issue of the *Grown-Up Persons' Home Journal* or *Not for Men Only,* this month featuring the Eat Only Between Meals Diet or the Ten Pounds Off in Nine Days Diet, simply would not sell.

This is one unfortunate and painful fact that any serious approach to attaining a healthy body weight must not ignore: There is no easy way. If you think that somewhere one exists, forget it. There ain't no such animal! Real growth and change are never painless or without difficulties.

You have been taught the opposite in many ways, chiefly by the advertising agencies. Again and again you have been told that if you do one simple thing (after buying their product) all your problems will be solved. If you put a dab of "Forbidden" deodorant under your armpits you will become irresistible to the opposite sex and will soon be wearing perfectly fitting evening clothes as you drive up to a very fancy party in your convertible. (And the weather will, of course, be perfect!) Eat Wheaties and become a champion. Of what is unspecified—after all it's your fantasy!

Before we go further with this, there is a general attitude to discuss. I know of no better way to put this than in the famous four rules that Barry Commoner used to describe the basic laws of ecology. They are:

1. Everything is connected to everything else.

2. Everything must go somewhere.

3. Mother Nature knows best.

4. There is no free lunch.

These rules apply as well to the individual person as they do to ecological systems. Looked at in reverse order they tell you that you attain no real growth and development without work and effort, that the more you treat, feed, and use your body and being in the ways you are built for, the better it will be; that the results of your problems will always eventually surface somewhere; and that you cannot "fix" one system of your being on any permanent basis without its affecting and continuing to be affected by other systems. You function as a whole in an environment, and the natural ways are the best, but to reach them you will probably have to work pretty hard.

One set of problems arises from your own feelings about your weight. Over and over again, people with weight problems who are in psychotherapy have come to recognize all kinds of crazy belief systems they were not even aware they had subscribed to. Some believed that if they were thin enough all their sexual problems would be solved. I have seen people, far past adolescence, who weighed less than one hundred pounds who still believed they could solve their problems by losing weight. Other anorectics and bulimics have exactly the opposite craziness—they believed that if they were thin enough, they would have no sexual characteristics and therefore be safe from their own impulses.

People who are seriously overweight may well be dealing with similar unconscious beliefs. Some feel that as long as they are fat they are safe from their sexuality. Others see being fat as a way of holding back their own anger at this or that situation or person. Or, perhaps as punishing someone or themselves. The fact that these beliefs are often unconscious does not lessen their effect on us. They can be very powerful forces leading to a great deal of self-sabotage.

Very often, as we really begin to work toward a healthy body weight, these fantasies surface and we become very conscious of them. If you are working with a good psychotherapist, this certainly gives you some good material to talk about. If you are in a group where it is appropriate to discuss this, you will probably be surprised by the number of others who share your feelings.

Suppose, however, that neither of these situations exists and that there is simply no one you can discuss your feelings with. Then I suggest you remember an old teaching of the psychiatrist William Alanson White and apply it. He said somewhere that nearly all of us are pretty normal in most areas of our existence and that all of us are pretty neurotic or eccentric (depending on how wealthy we are) in a couple of areas. Further, each of us has one area in which we are complete fruitcakes—one area of our existence in which we are completely crazy. It is one of the tasks of adulthood, said White, to determine what that area is and either cure ourselves of it or accept it and compensate for it. So, therefore, if you do discover your own particular craziness, recognize it, smile at it when you can, and do your damnedest to compensate for it.

A SECOND SET of problems comes from the attitudes and behaviors of other people. Frequently the very people who have been bugging you for years to lose weight, now that you are seriously on the road, begin to sabotage you in one way or another. This is something more that you will have to deal with in whatever way you personally find effective, but do expect it. Mostly it comes from *their* fantasies and from the fact that most people do not like to think. When someone they care about changes, they have to think, and unconsciously they try to push that person back into the old way of being so that they can continue to react to him automatically and not have to think in new ways. The following is a group of observations Eda LeShan made on examples of this in her book *Winning the Losing Battle.**

> We have had a series of visitors recently and it suddenly occurred to me that in the past several months we have received salt and pepper sets as gifts from three different people. That's more than I have gotten in my thirty-four years of marriage! And all since I announced to the world that I'd be on a salt-free diet for the rest of my life! Weird.
>
> Maxine wrote me about adjusting to being back home. She listed the comments she's been hearing. "A self-righteous aunt said, 'You better keep it off!' A friend who can't stop smoking said, 'You're much too thin now.' From a fat friend whose husband had just complimented me: 'It's just as dangerous to be too thin as to be too fat.' A friend at the golf course said, 'It's great while it lasts, but I never met anyone who didn't gain it all back.' It's wonderful to be home!"
>
> I got an emergency call—would I come and give a speech in Chicago? Pat got stuck at the last minute and is desperate. When I said no, I was still dieting and traveling was just too difficult, she said in a slightly patronizing tone, "Well, I wouldn't want to do anything to interfere with your health, but you're not sick—are you just doing this for beauty?"
>
> I called New York on business this morning and Bill's secretary was feeling very chatty. "We all love you just the way you are," she told me. "You shouldn't deprive yourself of the pleasures of food—life is too short. It's not necessary to be thin at your age." She's thirty and wears a size 5!

* New York: Thomas Crowell, 1979.

I met Dan quite by accident in an airport the other day. He yelled at me, "There's less of you to love!" I wanted to kill him on the spot. I said, "Don't you ever dare say that to me again—you of all people, who chase every broad who looks like Twiggy!" He left hurriedly. I don't think we will be likely to have any further conversations!

Last night Diane called to find out how I was doing. I told her I had lost thirty pounds. Her first comment was, "How will I know you?" That's a terrifying question, which plays right into my own anxieties. But that was minor; then she said, "Poor Larry, all the men will be chasing after you!" The implication was clear that while I was fat, there was no such danger.

Roger wrote me: "Why did you have to go to North Carolina to starve to death? You could have done it at home and all your friends could have witnessed your disappearance." Thin people seem to have some of the same fantasies fat people have!

Letter from Kate: "I don't like the idea of your being skinny. You might look gaunt and less inviting and warm."

Alice called. She said, "I'll be so jealous! Now you'll be famous and successful and thin! It's almost too much to bear!"

Nadine came back from a visit home. She reported to us how it felt to be among "civilians" again. Not good, "Everybody congratulated me and complimented me, but nobody believed I was really serious about staying thin. People were constantly inviting me out to lunch and dinner and to cocktail parties. They kept trying to entice me to have 'just one tiny drink,' or 'You must just taste this.' The world is full of saboteurs," she told us.

⌇

ONE OF THE things to decide early on when you are setting up a program is whether you want to get healthy or to get thin. These are not the same thing. "Thin" refers chiefly to your appearance, to how others see you. If you want to spend your life working on this, fine! Someday you are likely to grow up and then you will shift to "healthy," which refers chiefly to how you judge yourself and how much zest and enjoyment you are getting out of life. It is certainly true that many of us have to change our body weight in order to become more healthy, to enjoy ourselves and our life more, and to have a better chance of avoiding many diseases. To be healthy, you need an exercise system as well as an adjustment of your eating habits.

Do not confuse "work" with "exercise." You may do a tremendous amount of work and be exhausted at the end of the day, but unless at some time during the day you work your muscles hard you are not using them fully, and unless at some time you work your cardiovascular system and increase its level of activity for a solid period of time, you are not using it fully, and you are not very likely to increase the function of either. Exercise works the muscular and/or cardiovascular systems hard. It leaves you wanting to rest and (unless you are swimming) perspired.

An exercise program is essential for health but not for thinness. (Concentration camp inmates were very thin, but certainly not healthy!) You cannot meditate a fit muscle system or a healthy cardiovascular system no matter how hard you try. And these are a part of you and necessary for a healthy body weight—for a healthy body.

There are no rules about how to devise a "good" exercise program. People differ so much in so many ways that any rule would have more exceptions than it would have people who should follow it. There *are* some good rules of thumb—aspects to consider. Do it on a regular basis—three, four, or five times a week. Do not strain yourself to exhaustion—set up a program that will leave you feeling pleasantly tired. Find a type of exercise that you enjoy or at least do not find actively unpleasant. Once you have set up your program follow it with as much discipline and rigor as you can—you have made a promise to yourself and you will like yourself much more if you keep it than if you do not. By and large, most people trying to adjust their weight should avoid weight lifting and Nautilus-type equipment. You are trying to reintegrate the whole body and mind into one well-functioning whole, not just to build up bulky muscles. But here also there are exceptions. You may well be one of them!

MAUREEN HAD NEVER had a weight problem until her husband walked out on her when she was in her late forties. She had been raised in New York City, lived in her parents' home while she went to Columbia University where she studied liberal arts, and then, on graduation, moved directly into her new home with her brand-new husband. She spent the next twenty years keeping house, raising two children, and encouraging his career. She worked hard to help him succeed, scrimping and pinching pennies so that they would have more money to invest in his company. Finally the business began to succeed and then, rather suddenly, became extremely profitable, and they were quite well off. They put money into a college fund for the children, moved into a much nicer apartment, and then, one Sunday morning he got up, told her he was moving in with another—younger—woman, and left. For the next two years, Maureen felt completely lost and extremely sorry for herself. She had enough alimony not to have to work. She went to plays, an occasional art museum, a lot of movies, and saw friends until they became tired of commiserating with her. In the first year she gained fifty pounds, in the second she gained twenty more.

At the end of the second year she felt completely desperate and knew she had to do something about the situation or she would eat herself into the grave. She began to look for a psychotherapist. She was intelligent enough to know that in spite of her real need she had to find the right person and began the necessary "shopping" that everyone has to go through today to locate a therapist with whom they can work. The first five she saw all had well-furnished offices in excellent locations and fairly full schedules. They were well dressed, well mannered, and had impressive diplomas and licenses hanging on their walls. She realized that not one of them saw her as an individual, an adult who had suffered and striven and done her best, but all of them saw her as a fat woman whom they knew how to fix with the same technique they used with everyone they saw. They all had been trained to believe that there is one way to "do" psychotherapy (although they disagreed on exactly what that method was), and that if they applied it correctly to everyone who came into their office they would help everyone who was treatable—and it was just unfortunate that the rest were not. She saw each of these for one session and looked further.

The sixth therapist she tried was quite different. After the session she called a friend and said, "She's wonderful. She's not trying to fix me but to help me become more myself. And she thinks that would be something special. I think that maybe she's nuts, but I like her and she likes me. In any case, she's the first one I've seen who knows I'm a real person and not just a member of 'the class of fat women who need my help, poor things'!"

Maureen worked with this therapist for about a year and

felt much better about her life. She began to go more regularly to museums and to take courses in art history at a nearby university. Presently she was accepted into a training course for docents at the Metropolitan Museum of Art. After the initial training, she was assigned groups to lead through special sections of the museum, lecturing to them on the artists and their paintings. She discovered that she enjoyed this tremendously and looked forward to getting up in the morning and going to work. As she found life more interesting, other people found her more interesting. She had more to talk about than how unfair life had been to her and how hard it was. Her social life improved.

The only problem she could not seem to deal with successfully was her weight. Although she explored many facets of this problem in psychotherapy—her fear of how she would behave if she were thin and attractive, her need to punish herself for what had happened to her, and so forth—she simply could not get a real grip on attaining her best and healthiest body weight. She tried a few groups such as Overeaters Anonymous but did not feel that they were right for her. Two weeks at a luxurious weight loss center were delightful; she loved being pampered and massaged and generally taken care of. She lost ten pounds, but regained them within the next few weeks. She agreed with her therapist that even if she could afford to stay in the spa for the rest of her life, it would not solve any real problems. She knew that ultimately she had to do it for herself if she were to maintain the weight loss. She decided to try the meditation route. For her program, she chose the Contemplation meditation and used a seashell to work with. After the five-week period she had decided on, she gave it up and went instead to Breath Counting with which she felt much more at home. For the second basic meditation she chose the Thousand Petal Lotus with the word "food" in the center. She stayed with this for the entire time she worked with the program. She found that it helped her to really comprehend one of the things she had been discussing in her psychotherapy: that no part of her was separate from any other part; that her history and her feelings and her physiology all interacted and that it was not possible to really draw a sharp line among them; that each was a different aspect of her total being; that Maureen functioned as a whole, not as a collection of parts. She also started to one-point her breakfasts and found that she began to want less food and to move gradually toward a much healthier diet in the mornings. Later she discovered the same process taking place for her eating during the rest of the day.

During the ninth week of her program Maureen went to a movie and just before it started saw her ex-husband and his new wife sitting six rows ahead of her. They were laughing together and holding hands and seemed to be having a wonderful time. She was terribly upset, all the old feelings of being sorry for herself returned. At two o'clock in the morning she was still awake, got out of bed, got dressed, and took a taxi to an all-night grocery store ten blocks away.

She brought home two large paper bags full of all kinds of junk food. As she spread her purchases out on the kitchen table, the sheer amount of food startled her. She looked at the opened box of Oreos (she had eaten half a dozen on the way home) and decided to try to delay further bingeing for a few moments. She did a hard ten minutes of Breath Counting during which she made the strongest effort she could to stay with the exercise and bring her mind back to the counting as soon as it wandered off. At the end of the alotted time, she looked again at the mountain of food on the table, laughed at herself, and swore that her ex-husband was no longer going to run her life. She threw the rest of the Oreos down the incinerator and put all the unopened food into a large plastic bag, which she took the next morning to a nearby soup kitchen for the homeless. Her self-confidence was markedly increased by this incident, but just in case, she decided to add a mantra to her program for the next month. She chose "I am in charge of my life" and stayed with it for the period she had promised herself. After that she did not feel any need to continue it.

After a good deal of thought and some experimentation, she chose an exercise program to go with the meditation. This consisted of going to a local gymnasium three times a week and simply walking at a steady pace on a treadmill. She did not try to run or exhaust herself or anything like that, but over the first ten minutes, she gradually increased the speed of the treadmill to three miles an hour and stayed there for forty minutes. She then gradually decreased the speed, ending at a slow walk of two miles an hour. At her therapist's suggestion, she has made the central forty minutes into a meditation in which she simply tries to be aware of what she is doing—walking—and of nothing else. (This is an exercise used very much by the self-development school known as the Gurdjieff Work and can be very good for some people. Others tend to develop an unpleasant sense that it is not right for them. Those for whom this happens should, of course, give it up.) For Maureen it was a good exercise and felt very much right in spite of the frequent periods during which her mind obstinately wandered all over the place. After the treadmill, she would have a massage or sit for a few minutes in the steam room, then shower and rest for an hour. This way of taking care of herself usually made her feel very good and she slept exceptionally well those nights.

During the next year, there were three more occasions when emotions and outside events combined to make it difficult for Maureen to continue her program. On two of those occasions she ate herself into exhaustion. After each of these she went back to the mantra for a month. More importantly, however, she had learned not to attack herself when this happened, but to smile at herself for having the weaknesses and problems that come with being human, and to recognize that she had tried, was trying very hard, and really deserved to take pride in her ability to keep trying, not to criticize herself for her weakness and human fraility.

At this writing, Maureen been on the program for over a year. She is close to the weight she would like to maintain and feels good about herself and her life. She has a boyfriend who seems to be getting pretty serious, but she is far from ready to marry him. "He's okay and a lot of fun," she says. "But he's really not up to my level!"

# ·5·

≈

# Special Problems in Meditation

*T*HE FIRST AND most widespread problem reported by people who are using meditation is that they simply cannot do it. They say they cannot meditate because their mind constantly wanders and it is impossible for them to concentrate. When they do achieve concentration briefly, they cannot sustain it. Over and over again I have heard this from people who are trying to learn to meditate. Frequently they give up in despair and say that they just cannot learn to do it right. "No matter how hard I work," they have frequently told me, "my mind keeps wandering off. I cannot keep my mind on the exercise as I am supposed to. I guess it's just not for me." And they quit.

People who react in this way think they are different from others. They think that some or most other people or nearly everyone else *can* meditate without constant distraction, without constantly wandering off and losing the focus of what they are doing. This idea is completely wrong!

*"No one learns to meditate well."* No one. Not even those mythical "perfect masters" one hears about in the New Age movement. St. Theresa of Avila was once told by one of her novices that it must be wonderful to be like her and not

constantly bothered by mental and emotional disturbances during her devotions. Theresa replied, "What do you think I am, a Saint?" St. Bernard, who knew a great deal about these matters, was once asked how often during his meditations he was just doing them and nothing else, his mind was not wandering off. With a sigh that still echoes down these long centuries he replied, "How rare the hour and how brief its duration!" Mystics and students of meditation in the East do not do any better, but they are much less likely to admit it.

It is something similar to walking for exercise. We all do it at about the same level of skill, although some may be a bit better than others; but not much. Some people, however, do it more consistently than others. Some do it as part of a health program specifically adapted to *their* needs rather than just as an exercise they took off the rack in the store, one that fits everyone more or less and no one really well. These people—those who do it consistently and as part of a program designed for them—get better results than others. But they do not "walk better" or become much more expert at walking. They just do it more consistently and as part of a program so that their *results* are better than the results achieved by those who do not do these things.

How does your meditational practice change with experience? First, you learn to catch yourself more quickly when you drift off and to bring yourself back to the work more firmly, lovingly, gently. You learn to work more consistently. You learn to smile more indulgently at your resistances to the work as you encounter them and deal with them. Eventually you also learn that you feel better when you do your regular program of meditation and miss it when you skip it. This provides some extra motivation to keep it up on a regular basis.

As you practice, don't you get better? Don't you have longer and longer periods of just "doing them," of being

awake, aware, alert and just being conscious of one thing—
the meditation? The answer here is a clear and unqualified
"sometimes." Probably, over time, your development will be
toward a pattern that is more and more erratic and extreme.
During some sessions there will be serious and definite periods when you are really "into it." These are the sessions
when for solid portions of the time you are really completely
following the directions you gave yourself at the beginning.
You come out of one of these with a sort of "wow!" feeling—
a sense of having really "gotten into it!" of being sort of
"charged up" and perhaps also pleasantly relaxed and gently
fatigued. Then there will be sessions at the opposite end of
the spectrum. Sessions in which your mind simply seems to
refuse to stay on any one subject and wanders madly all over
the place like a top spinning rapidly out of control and wob-
bling around like three extremely drunken passengers on a
pitching ocean liner. The analogy may sound overblown and
extreme, but that is certainly the way it feels sometimes. You
come out of these sessions with a feeling of frustration, but—
if you have stayed with it the full period and kept working at
it—you also feel good, somehow stronger, with an increased
sense of your ability to cope with problems. Sort of an "Oh
boy, if I can stay with a session like that and not be thrown
by it, it's going to take an awful lot to defeat me. I'm tougher
and more competent than I thought." If, however, you have
just given up in the middle when the session seemed to go so
crazy, you will have less confidence in yourself and the future. You will feel much less good about yourself.

One pattern that develops in many meditational programs, just as you feel you are getting the hang of it and
learning how to stay with it, is a period where all the meaning and purpose seem to go out of your program. Emotionally you find yourself unable to connect with the reason you
are doing it. The juice goes out of the work and it simply

seems tedious and meaningless. (To use an old American phrase—you find yourself up to the waist in alligators and can't remember why you are clearing the swamp!)

Thomas Merton, the Trappist monk who made a deep and many years' study of meditation (I recommend in particular his book *The Ascent to Truth),* wrote of these times that during them you feel as if your mind and emotions were full of dry dust.

If when this occurs you put your head down, remember your promise to yourself, and follow your commitment, the feeling will pass fairly quickly. If you don't, if you stop in order to give the feeling time to dissipate, or if you start trying gimmicks to jump-start your work, it will wreck your entire program.

If I seem to be saying that meditation is a grim and unpleasant business, this is not so. It is an exciting and fulfilling adventure. But, as in any real adventure, there are tough times and traps. If you know about these in advance, you will be much more able to handle and override them when and if you meet them, and you are likely to have a far more interesting and enjoyable voyage. I would not be writing this book, nor would I have stayed involved in the study of meditation all these many years, if I did not know that for most people it can provide a useful and fascinating way to deal with many problems and to help us get on with our basic problem of learning, all our life, to live more fully, richly, and zestfully. The game is well worth the candle!

So, to end this discussion of a particular problem—if you feel (as you are very likely to from time to time) that you cannot meditate well, you are right. But neither can anyone else! Do not expect to learn to meditate well and do not expect to get much better as you progress, any more than you would expect to get somewhere riding a stationary bicycle in the gymnasium. You won't, but the working at it is good for you and that's the reason you are doing it!

The second most frequent problem in meditational programs is what I call the "I just don't have the time" syndrome. This is frequently amplified as "I lead a busy and complicated life and I just can't manage the extra half-hour a day. After all I have to earn my living, and/or take care of the kids, and/or get to all the places on my schedule each day, and/or make sure my clothes are ready for tomorrow, and/or . . . and so forth." This is often felt and presented as "I was doing all right until the boss gave me the extra assignment and the kids got chicken pox and the refrigerator broke down and my car pool disbanded" . . . and etc., and etc.

Yes, it is often difficult for most of us to find that extra half-hour or so a day that we can use to really take care of ourselves. The demands of the outside world—outside of our consciousness that is—are often heavy and complex. Before you start a meditation program you should be clear about your priorities. Just how important is attaining a healthy body weight? Take a few minutes and really look at that question. Is it important enough to assign a half-hour a day to it and then to keep the promise? If not, *do not start.*

Certainly there are real emergencies. I wrote in Chapter 1 that when these are of the caliber that require the firefighters or paramedics arriving at your door the emergency takes precedence. But short of this level of disaster, you and I know that we can always somehow find the necessary half-hour if we regard our weight and health as important. How important? You have to decide this for yourself. I can only tell you in advance that one of the most common resistances to meditation is the feeling that you are overwhelmed by the pressure of external events and demands and cannot find the time or energy to take care of yourself. Further, I can say on the basis of long personal experience, and also of experience with teaching meditation, that if you give in to this feeling (short of the firefighters-paramedics level of disaster), it will be more and more often too hard to find the time and you will eventually lose the program entirely. If, however, you make the time, even if you have to do your program late at night when you are exhausted, the time and energy will begin to "appear" and will become easier and easier to find as the days go on. Long experience has taught us that this is the best way to deal with the problem. And that for people starting a meditation program, it is indeed a widespread stumbling block.

Another problem that frequently appears when using a meditation program to achieve a specific purpose—such as reaching a healthy body weight—is the belief that you are not "ready" to do it. You say to yourself, in effect, "I have too many unfinished problems from my childhood to really take care of myself." This takes many specific forms. "I cannot get my weight to a healthy level because I unconsciously do not believe that I deserve it." Or "I must stay overweight so that I remain unattractive to the opposite sex." Or "I must not lose weight as it is the extra weight that helps me keep my unacceptable emotions in check." Or other variations on this theme.

All or any of these may be unconscious reasons for having sabotaged past weight loss programs and for doing the same thing again. If the feelings are too strong for you to handle by will and determination, you may need a psychotherapy program to help you out. But sooner or later you are going to have to take control—decide who is running your life, you as you are now or unconscious feelings from your childhood. When you make the decision that it must be you as you are at this time, you will be ready to do the job!

(All of the above applies, of course, to the unconscious

crazinesses that make you too thin as well as those that make you too fat. Both are equally neurotic drives.)

It is true that "willpower" is a very unpopular term today in sophisticated as well as in psychological and psychiatric circles. This is, in large part, a reaction to its overuse in the last century and the earlier part of this one. In some groups, however, this aversion has been taken to a pretty ridiculous extreme. (It is not true that they immediately throw you out of whatever school of psychotherapy you are in if they catch you talking about willpower, but you are certainly likely to flunk the specific course in which you mentioned it! And get sent back for more psychotherapy yourself!)

There are times, however, when it is necessary to say, "I am the boss of me—not my childhood experiences," and then to act as if this is so. The notion that you are helpless in the face of your neurotic drives is an easy and a popular one today, but it has probably helped lead you to the position you are now in if you are reading this book. It is time to discard it in favor of a better idea!

Certainly it is wise, before starting any new program involving your physical body, to check with your physician. There may be a medical problem that affects your body weight. Checking out your physiology is, however, a far cry from not solving the weight problem because of emotional needs. Make sure there is not an endocrinogical or other physical factor at work—you may, as one example, need thyroid medication—then, having cleared this, get to work.

⌒

ANOTHER CLASS OF special problems related to attaining a healthy body weight lies in those special times when we rest and relax from our normal routines. "I was doing fine with the program until I went on the cruise [on vacation, to the hotel, etc.] where they served meals five times a day and everyone was always eating, and the food was already paid for, and it was served so attractively," etc. Or "The program was running well until my friends [relatives, etc.] came to visit, and we spent so much time at the table talking, and they wanted to go out to dinner every other night," etc. There are other variations on this theme, but you will recognize them and can choose the ones that most apply to you.

Let us look at these oh-so-plausible statements. Translated into honest English they say, "I let other people and external circumstances choose my eating habits and dictate how I treat my body and myself. I take offered opportunities to give up this pesky diet and this meditation program." Put this way, these statements are far less plausible. They sound much more like what they actually are—excuses.

A cruise or a vacation is a time for *you*. You are not working to support the family or to build up your retirement fund or to pay off the mortgage, to fill your children's college funds, or what have you. It is for you, and you can decide in advance that this time will be used for the best aspects and parts of you. It is a time to catch up on sleep, exercise, vegetative needs, and perhaps junky novels, to breathe fresh air, see new sights, do new things, perhaps get new ideas. It is a time to increase your real positive forces and abilities and not, as you have probably done in the past, to reinforce negative ones.

You will be aware in advance if and when you are going on vacation and (usually) if friends or relatives are coming to visit. Before this happens—two weeks or more in advance—act as if you are in a stress period. Add one of the meditations from Chapter 4 to your program. Then, during the vacation or visit, *keep up the program*. There will almost always be time if you act as if you require it. It will increase your good feelings about yourself and your self-confidence if you actively carry out the program through the vacation.

It is not necessary to be extreme or exhibitionistic about this. Taste the good food served in the cruise ship dining room or in your relative's favorite restaurant if you wish. But keep the portions small. You will find the delectables just as satisfying if you eat one spoonful as you will if you empty the entire plate. And if you eat only the one or two spoonsful, you will be far more satisfied with yourself and enjoy the cruise much more. Adlai Stevenson used to tell the story of the little girl in school who was asked if she knew how to spell "banana." She answered, "I know how to spell it, but I never know when to stop." When trying to achieve your own healthy body weight, follow the general rule of stopping early in the course of each dish. You will feel a lot better that way!

What I have been writing about here also applies, of course, to those times when you are under heavy emotional pressure. You are suddenly informed that a neighbor with whom you have had what you believed to be a long, good, and loving relationship is suing for a portion of your land on the grounds that she often parked her car there and that, therefore, she now owns it by right of adverse possession. Or you are told that three out of four of the people in your department will be fired in one month and that in thirty days you will be informed if you are one of the three or if you are the lucky fourth; or your son is arrested for dealing drugs in Cleveland, where you thought he was going to college and about to get his engineering degree. Or your company downsized last year and your job of twenty-three years vanished and there appear to be no jobs available in the country for which you are not either underqualified or overqualified.

This type of disaster strikes us all at one time or another. They and their like are real, extremely painful, and deeply disturbing. It is easy and natural at such times to say, in effect, "I have had it. I have so much to worry about and to take care of that I simply do not have the time or energy to go on with this silly meditation or with this dieting. At least I can have the pleasure of food until things quiet down, and then if they ever do and I'm still alive I'll get back to work."

The translation of this is that things are so difficult and painful that you are going to give up what control you still have of your own destiny and join whatever forces there are in the universe that seem bent on destroying you. You are saying that since things seem to be against you, you are going to join in and be against your own health and what remains of your sense of well-being and autonomy. To make this plain, which would *really* give you more pleasure—the extra portion and the dessert at dinner with the ice cream snack at bedtime, or the knowledge that "they" have not been able to defeat you, that you are still in there fighting and moving toward your own best health and good feeling? The taste and the memory of that hot fudge sundae will quickly fade; the good feeling you get from staying with your program will last far longer. And it will be a far greater aid in whatever struggle with the world you are in at this and in future times.

The hardest times are those when we are in deep grief for someone we love. We get through these periods best by accepting our grief and sadness and hurt. Each of us, of course, does best by expressing it in his own way, and these range from keeping a stiff upper lip to letting others see us weep. However, there is one thing that we all can do at these times —ask ourselves what the people we have lost would want for us. Would they want their death to make us less and destroy us or would they want us to go on to a fuller growth and development? Would they wish for us more or less growth, more or less of our giving in to our neurotic patterns; our gaining in health, or the reverse. Then, understanding the answers to these questions, we can try to use our love for them to fulfill what would have been their wishes for us in these terribly hard and painful times.

⌒

HERBERT AND DAVID SPIEGEL have done a good deal of work in the area of psychological treatment of various disorders. In their important book *Trance and Treatment\** they offer two excellent guidelines for attaining a healthy body weight.

> *The first guideline is this: always, always, eat with respect, with respect for your body. Because if you respect your body you are never likely to regard it as a garbage can. The more important part of that perspective is that you avoid the biggest trap of all, which is to tell yourself "Don't eat that." Once you get caught in that trap you are losing. It is like telling yourself, "Don't have an itch on your nose." Do you feel it? Or, "Try to think about not swallowing." Free people don't like to be told "don't." When God said to Adam and Eve, "Don't eat the apple," that was the end of Paradise. This is a basic observation about the human condition. Why not use this knowledge if you want to devise a strategy that can work? You can use it this way: turn it around and you have a corollary, which is that a far more effective way to change behavior is to do it on the basis of something you are for. So if you approach it this way, you will respect and protect your body. In the course of protecting your body from overeating you can radically change your behavior, but you feel it as "Yes, I respect my body" instead of "Don't eat that."*
>
> *The second of these two guidelines is going to surprise you. Learn to eat like a gourmet. Why a gourmet? Because a gourmet pays full attention to every swallow.*

\* *Washington, D.C.: American Psychiatric Press, 1978.*

*Every swallow is a total encounter with food. He is
aware of the touch, the taste, the smell, the temperature,
the texture of the food, and with such total involvement
that it is incredible how much fulfillment and enjoyment
he gets out of each swallow. In fact, this whole process
not only helps you to radically change your eating behavior, but it brings joy back to eating again. The gourmet does not make the mistake of saying, "Oh I swal-
lowed that food, but I don't remember what it tastes like,
I had better take another bite." The reason a gourmet
does not make that mistake is because each swallow is
such a total involvement that the memory of it stays with
him. He doesn't have to keep getting reinforcements of
new food because he knows fully what the experience
was. The stereotype that gourmets are overweight is just
not true. Most of the great gourmets of the world are
either of normal weight or are underweight.*

These two guidelines clearly work in the same direction
as the meditational program offered in this book. The similarity, for example, of the second and the meditation of one-
pointing one meal a day is obvious.

# ·6·

≈

## Individualizing Your
## Weight Control Program

ALL THROUGH THIS book I
have been stressing, and will continue to stress, the need to
individualize your program. For it to be most effective it
must be one that is uniquely yours and not one that you
have "taken off the rack." Your fingerprints and your retinal
patterns and your body chemistry and your genetic inheri-
tance and your life experiences are unique and like no one
else's. Similarly, a program to achieve a healthy body weight
should be one of a kind. I have given choices as to the
meditations you can use to design the best program for you
without giving so many that you would be overwhelmed
with indecision. Further, there is nothing sacrosanct or written in stone about any specific meditation except the discipline of really working to be doing one thing at a time and of
keeping your promises to yourself by staying with whatever
exact form you have chosen for the period you have decided
on. I have given the forms that, after some experimentation, I
believe to be best for the widest variety of people today, but
if you are Breath Counting and wish to count your exhalations *and* your inhalations, or count up to ten instead of up
to four, Fine! Choose the form you will do and decide how

long each session will be, and how many weeks the next
period of work will be, and then follow through. At the end
of the full period, reevaluate, perhaps experiment a bit more
if you wish, and then you are off again on the next ride!

We have learned the importance of this in meditation
through long experience. There is no right way to meditate
that applies to everyone. Each person must find his own
exact forms. One of the reasons that there are so many "fail-
ures" in meditation is that most meditational schools and
teachers believe there is one right way for everyone and that,
by a curious coincidence, it is the one they have learned from
their teacher and from their school! It may in fact *be* the best
way for them as individuals, but it is not right for everyone,
and so many people, after experimenting with it will realize
that there is something wrong, and leave the program. These
people then believe that they have tried meditation and that
it did not work for them, and generally they do not return
and try other meditational paths.

There are certain basic aspects that are central to all serious meditational programs. Constantly striving for "one-
pointing" for "bare attention" (in some schools it is called
"coherent attention"), that is, disciplining of the mind to do
one thing at a time; keeping one's promises to oneself; learning to treat oneself in a loving but demanding-the-best manner, these are constants. Beyond that, specific forms, or
whether you work sitting in an armchair or in a lotus position with your legs crossed over each other, or lying comfortably on a floor, or squatting in a shaman's position, or walking in a peaceful area, or whatnot, are up to you. You should
decide whether it will be best for you to work once a day,
twice a day, four, five, six, or seven times a week and for
periods of anything from four to eight weeks as a specific
promise to yourself.

As you proceed, if you decide to go beyond your work to

achieve a healthy body weight and to design a meditational program for your best general development, you may find that it is best for you to work on any one of a number of different meditational paths, or on a specially chosen combination. For example there are paths of physical meditation such as Hatha Yoga, Sensory Awareness (the Gindler Method), Tai Chi, or the Alexander Method. There are paths of meditation that stress work through the emotions such as Bhakti Yoga and various of the forms devised in Western religious groups. There are forms of meditational work that stress the intellectual path such as Ynana Yoga, the Gurdjieff Work, Habad Hassidism, and others. There are paths that stress meditation through certain attitudes during work such as Karma Yoga, the Little Way of St. Thérèse of Lisieux, the Way of Action, and others. Anyone wishing to use the meditational path for long term and general development should look at these possibilities and choose the one, or the combination of ones, that are best for him or her as a unique and one-of-a-kind individual.

Whatever path you choose to use to grow and change toward fulfilling your individual potential will, unfortunately, require hard and long work. There is no easy road. Change and growth are very difficult. They take serious and continued effort.

This seems rather strongly put, but those of us who have made serious attempts to change and grow past where we are now will attest to its truth. In working to achieve a healthy body weight, it is not only our meditational work that we need to individualize, it is the other aspects of our work in this direction also. Let us look at a few of these.

I wrote in Chapter 1 about the need to choose a diet that fits you and is not simply the popular diet of the moment. Find a nutritionist if you wish, but choose one who will not decide on the correct diet before discussing with you your past eating habits, what foods give you energy and do not cause you to "crash" afterward, what foods are addictive for you so that once you start eating them you continue to want more and more until you are stuffed and but still feel unsatisfied, etc. Further, there should be discussion of the best eating patterns for you—are you naturally a three-meal-a-day person, a two, a four-meal-a-day, a "snacker" who nibbles all day, or what? I once sent a friend with a severe heart condition to a nutritionist. This friend was one of those people who is pretty unfocused for the first few hours each day. She worked at home, and in the morning before going to her office down the hall to see her first client, it was all she could do to turn on the light under the coffee she had prepared the previous night and she would stand there sort of swaying while it heated. Since she was highly motivated to diet, she could also have, if it were prescribed, taken some juice or fruit out of the refrigerator or even forced herself to make some toast or cold cereal. The nutritionist prescribed a very good diet for her condition, but one that would have required her to juice and grind and blend various concoctions fresh for her breakfast each day. The diet was simply irrelevant for this particular person. It may have been theoretically right for her condition, but the nutritionist forgot that she was not treating a condition, but a specific person with a condition. This is a somewhat extreme example, but the majority of diets do not work because they are designed for a group of people in general and there are no individual people in general. They are all specific!

There are, of course, general rules for dieting which include such things as calories, cholesterol, and so on. These are important to know, and a nutritionist can be a real help. But you can probably do the job yourself with a little careful reading. (Read serious material. Ignore all diets invented or recommended by the *National Enquirer* and such like.) But the main thing is to check against your own experience, to try those things that make sense to you, and to see how they work. There is an ancient manuscript, the Kalama Sutra, which is usually believed to have been written by the Buddha. In part, it states:

> Do not believe on the strength of traditions even if they have been held in honor for many generations and in many places; do not believe anything because many people speak of it; do not believe on the strength of sagas of old times; do not believe that which you yourself have imagined thinking a God has inspired you. Believe nothing which depends on the authority of your masters or of priests. After investigation believe that which you yourself have tested, and which is for your good and that of others.

These are good rules to follow when choosing the elements of a program for your own health, development, and healthy body weight.

If your diet includes, as it well may, some vitamin or mineral supplements, again decide on the kind, amount, and frequency of intake on the basis of who you are and not on the basis of what is recommended in the popular or even the scientific journals. This seems so obvious that it should not be worth mentioning, but it is generally ignored. If I am six feet three inches and weigh 295 pounds when I start, and you are five feet one and weigh 160, it should be clear that the amount of vitamin C that would be right for you is not the same amount that would be right for me. And if I smoke, and live in a city where I inhale far more pollutants than you do, and you are on the pill, these are obvious factors for us both to take into account on our monthly trip to the health food store. However, strange as it may seem, most people ignore factors like these and decide on what supplements to add to their diet from the recommendations on the bottles, or because of something they have heard somewhere. And they take "standard" amounts of whatever they take and never worry about what that means or who decided on what standards are and for whom. These standards are often determined for reasons that have little to do with your individual health. Some years ago a study was made with a large number of physicians. They were sent two questionnaires several weeks apart. In the first, a lot of personal data was asked for, including their weight. In the second, they were asked for professional opinions, including the definition of "obesity." In nearly all cases they defined obesity as starting at a few pounds heavier than their own weight.

Various kinds of supplements can be a valuable addition to your diet, but choose them, preferably working together with someone who knows something about them, or else with a good book, on the basis of yourself and your lifestyle rather than on the basis some advertising specialist picked out of the air. And remember that when you are taking these additives, more is not necessarily better. A certain amount of vitamin A (for example) added to your daily intake can be very good for you and can help you in a number of ways. Too large an amount can land you in the hospital.

The importance of individualization at all levels cannot be overestimated and is generally underestimated. For many years now, the psychiatrist Herbert Spiegel has been trying to convince his colleagues in the health care profession that different patients need different kinds of psychotherapeutic help; that they need very different kinds of preparation for such stresses as surgery, and different kinds of help in dealing with grief, allergies, and what have you. His data is clear and his writing is scientific, readable, and has appeared in the most respectable journals as well as in his books. So strong, however, is the modern idea that what is sauce for the goose is sauce for the gander, that he has had little effect. Psychotherapists (like the teachers of meditation referred to earlier) nearly all believe that there is one correct method of psychotherapy for all patients and that it is the one they have learned at their teacher's knee. Both the efforts of colleagues like Spiegel and the efforts of their own patients to teach them otherwise are generally unsuccessful. Most people like things to be simple and it is far simpler to believe that there is only one correct path (whether we are dealing with psychotherapy, meditation, or anything else) than it is to face the complexity of everyone being different and to deal with the very real implication of this fact. Unfortunately for our comfort, however, everyone *is* different and this does have real implications.

The exercise and movement aspects of your program should also be individualized and designed for you rather than taken off the shelf of current best-sellers. If you are ready to add an exercise component to your program for achieving a healthy body weight, or to change the one you have been using, look around. What appeals to you? Find a type of exercise you would enjoy, one that leaves you with a good feeling after a session. It is conceivable that the popular one of the moment is the best one for you now. If so, go for it! But do not expect this to be so. If it happens, it is just coincidence. The range is very wide, and if it were not so frequently ignored, I would not find it necessary to write that you should take into account your general health, any specific medical conditions you happen to have, your previous exercise patterns, your age, and what your physician advises as your limits at this time. The potential range of exercises or combinations of exercises (there is no reason except popular prejudice that your exercise program should be made up of only one type of movement) is very large. It may well be that you will want to combine two or three for your specific program. Square dancing twice a week, swimming laps twice a week, and a long walk on Sundays is as reasonable a program as is jogging the same number of miles three or four mornings each week. You may find that working out five days a week on a rowing machine while you watch "The A Team" is your preferred mode at this time. Great! In five months you may change and find that a game of four-wall handball in the athletic club three times a week and a long swim on Wednesdays and Saturdays fits you now. Pick a program, stay with it a serious amount of time, and then reevaluate. You may decide to stay with it or to change. The important thing is that you listen to and observe who you are and what you need at this time in your life and development.

It should be clear from the above that, if you decide on a support group, an individual psychotherapist, or group therapy as part of your work, you should pick them carefully and in terms of what you need, not in terms of what local society, your local subculture, *Prevention* magazine, or the *New England Journal of Medicine* recommends!

In the sixteenth century, the sage Isaac Luria wrote, "There are six hundred thousand types of individuals. Each type has a different soul-root and needs a different type of nourishment in order to attain his or her fullest growth. It is the task of each person to find out which one of the six hundred thousand he or she is and thus to find the particular nourishment needed to reach their fullest being."

I do not know why Isaac Luria chose the particular number of six hundred thousand. I personally would say that there are as many types of individuals as there are individuals. Let us then each try to find the particular type of nourishment we need to attain our fullest growth. And to know that it will be different for each of us.

⌒

ONE FINAL NOTE on this subject. I have written over and over again that there is no right path for everyone. This includes meditation. It is an excellent way to solve problems for some people, a good way for the great majority, not relevant for some others. If, after seriously working at it for eight to sixteen weeks, you find that meditation is not for you, do not attack or criticize yourself on this ground. (If you do, it will only make your weight problem worse!) At the least, you will have had an adventure with your own mind and learned a good deal about yourself. You will have benefited from the experience even if meditation is not the right way for you to solve your weight problem.

There are a wide variety of factors in your genetic makeup and your life experiences that might place you in the "excellent," "good," or "irrelevant" category. The thing to do if, after serious work, you find that meditation is not for you is to explore some of the other avenues to solving your problems. These include psychotherapy (with the necessary shopping around that you will probably have to do), groups such as Overeaters Anonymous, spas, and upgrading your life in other areas in order to change your total ecology. Whatever adventure is right for you at this time in your development, Good Luck!

⌒

ELIZABETH, AT FORTY-SIX, was just as confused about her life as a teenager of thirteen—perhaps even more so. She married at eighteen, a man almost twice her age, whom she soon learned wanted a chattel, not a partner. The longer they lived together the more frightened she became. But she did not have the faintest idea that perhaps she had some choices; instead she gave birth to six children who became her husband's serfs. He was never physically abusive, but seemed to have enormous power over his family and others as well. He became a "business tycoon" by using the same aggressive persuasion, and Elizabeth figured she was lucky to have a mansion and a car and nice clothes. The only flaw in this was that with her children now mostly grown, she was shocked to discover that she had never lived and was a nonperson. This assessment began to occur to her on her fortieth birthday; with each succeeding year she gained an average of ten pounds. At forty-six she had a heart attack and discovered much to her amazement that she wanted to live.

At a health spa she managed to lose fifty pounds. At that point she realized that she hated to go home. Her husband was pleased with her new look and greeted her on her return with a list of social obligations, including having a dinner party for forty of his most intimate business associates.

Elizabeth promptly had a nervous breakdown, was hospitalized, and met a psychiatrist who told her, "You can't solve your problems by weight loss; the first priority is to figure out if you are a real person."

In the hospital, she began a meditation program. She did twenty minutes of Breath Counting each morning and one-pointed a meal once a day. She also chose to use a mantra. For this she chose the sentence "I am in charge of my life." She did the mantra for twenty minutes each morning and afternoon. In the morning she did it quietly, sitting in the dayroom. In the afternoon she did it more loudly, walking on the hospital grounds. For the first few weeks she could not seem to do it consistently, to follow the program every day. She kept "forgetting" or "something just came up just as I was starting." Then she gradually began to realize that she felt better, more put together and solid, on those days when she did the exercises than she did on those days when she omitted them. Gradually she became consistent and then very steady about them. After three months, she was not skipping any days at all.

She told her therapist that all her life people had been doing things to and for her. This, she said, included the hospitalization and, to a certain degree, the psychotherapy. The meditation program, she felt, was the first serious thing she had done to and for herself.

As an exercise program she chose a dancercize class offered at the hospital. She took this three times a week starting out at half an hour and then increasing it to an hour. After discharge from the hospital she continued the class at a studio near her home.

Elizabeth left the hospital, six months later. Shortly thereafter, she registered at a nearby college and divorced her husband. "I started to lose weight—very slowly—but steadily. By the time I got my degree in Early Childhood Education, I had figured out I existed! What a revelation! My problem was never about getting fat, it was discovering I had rights."

# ·7·

## Going On from There:
## Life After Dieting

*Y*OU HAVE NOW reached the place you set out for when you began this work. Or at least you recognize that you are well on the road. You have a meditation program in place that is helping you move toward a healthy body weight. Perhaps you have not reached it yet, but your adventure is well underway. Your confidence in yourself generally, and specifically in your ability to control your weight, increased markedly when you passed through some high-stress periods without dropping the program you had selected and promised yourself you would follow.

Now the time has come for the next step. The loss of weight-control that brought you to this book in the first place was not something that just "happened" to you. Life is not really like that, although it is simpler and easier to think that it is. Things don't just happen to us. We, as total human beings with physical, emotional, mental, and spiritual aspects, react to our total environment, from the temperature and pressure of the air to the behavior of others, and the general political climate we are in. There is, as the philosopher William James once remarked, no definite stopping place between a person's physiology and his philosophy. We are all of a piece; no part of us is separate from the others. Even when we are exposed to the bacteria or to the viruses of illness, how we react to them is determined not just by their virulence, but by the overall (and this includes the physical, mental, emotional, and spiritual aspects of our being) condition we are in. It is not only the virus, it is also the "terrain" on which it lands, as the physiologists of the late nineteenth century tried so hard to teach us. When I ask my physician, "Why did I catch this?" and get the reply, "There's a lot of it going around," I feel satisfied. It does not occur to me to ask why the next person on the train did not catch it, why one of the people I am living with caught it and not the others, or even why I did not catch it the last time there was "a lot of it going around." Every so often there appears a particularly virulent form of virus or bacteria—such as those of the great influenza epidemics that come from time to time as the pathogenic organism mutates into a new form—that tends to overwhelm our defenses and to resist the usual drugs and medications. But even when this happens (as in the various Asiatic flu epidemics or the great influenza disaster of 1918), the large majority of people do not get it. When the Black Plague ravaged Europe from the twelfth to the fifteenth centuries, and there were simply no preventive measures of any worth available, three quarters of the people did *not* catch it. The "terrain" was not right. Similarly, how we react to serious, stressful psychological events is determined not simply by the event itself, but by a synthesis of the event and the particular "terrain," that is, the total person involved.

For example, some years ago I was working in a child guidance clinic. In our catchment area a horrible incident occurred. Two hundred children were playing in a school yard. One nine-year-old girl ran out in the street to pick up a ball, looked up, and screamed loudly enough that every head in the yard turned just in time to see her run over and killed by a truck. Three weeks later one of the children from the school yard showed up at the clinic. Since the incident she had been unable to sleep, had thrown up after meals, and had repeated anxiety attacks. We all knew exactly what had caused these symptoms and were prepared to treat her on that basis. Then, in a staff conference, the chief of the clinic, Dr. Joseph Weinreb, asked us how many children from our area had witnessed the accident. When we replied "Two hundred," he asked, "Where are the other one hundred and ninety-nine?" Suddenly, we understood that a specific combination of trauma *and* terrain, interacting in this particular child, had led to the symptoms she experienced. Treatment, we saw, would have to be designed for a unique and individual person who had received a severe shock; it could not be an approach developed in terms of how one deals with the class of children who have received a severe shock.

To sum up, we each exist not as separate parts, but as a total human being who feels, thinks, acts, despairs or is enthusiastic, gets sick or stays well, is overweight or underweight, feels comfortable or ill at ease in the universe, is frightened or hopeful for the future, finds it difficult or finds it very difficult to change, and so forth.

Now that you are on the road to no longer being constantly concerned about your weight, it is time to look at the rest of your life. How much zest, enthusiasm, enjoyment do you experience in going about your daily rounds? Your body is now taking the shape you wish it to. Is your life doing the same? All the energy you have been putting into your weight problem—where could you now direct that energy to upgrade your life the most, to make it the most worthwhile and enjoyable?

We have arrived at the next stage of the program you started when you first read this book and decided to try the meditational path. Now that you are effectively dealing with that bothersome and painful weight problem, it is time to go on and improve the rest of your life. There is a real and good reason for including this chapter in a book on attaining a healthy body weight. If you wish to so change your total ecology that the combination of forces responsible for your weight problem is much less likely to reappear with the same unpleasant results, you will have to change other aspects of your life. If you do not, your victory in the weight area is likely to be short-lived. It is no accident that after so many successful diets, the people who worked so hard to succeed with them fall back and regain the weight or again become anorexic. These people did not go on to the next stage of the work, which was to so change their total being that those same forces could not reappear and overwhelm their good intentions once again.

There are two basic ways to do this. Before I describe them, however, it is important to point out that many people attempt to deal with recurring problems by using specific techniques or gimmicks. We learn to do this early in life, when we are taught such things as, "Count ten before you say anything when you are angry." We learn that when our heart starts pounding in frustration at an often repeated situation we should begin to breathe deeply or repeat a mantra or take a walk around the block. There are any number of these techniques that can be very useful in moments of frustration and/or rage. However, they do not do anything except deal with the tension of the moment that is threatening to explode inwardly or outwardly. They do nothing to prevent new situations of the same sort from happening. They do not change anything. If we wish to really change anything more than our feelings of the moment, we must use one of two basic methods. The first of these is to look at a specific problem, analyze its causes, find its sources, and thus deal with the problem as a real part of us, not simply as something that "happens." When we do this, we look at a problem in terms of our reactions, determine when we first began to react in this way, how we saw the world and ourselves at that time, and so forth. We try to see the kind of sense our actions made when we first adopted them and whether they still make sense in terms of our present view of who we are and what the world is like. This is the route of traditional psychotherapy; it is one of the greatest advances in understanding and one of the most wonderful tools for easing human suffering that we have ever known. It is sometimes an absolutely necessary method to use to solve certain problems.

This is the method designed by Sigmund Freud in the first part of the century. He also devised a specific way to go about it, but this is not used very much anymore and is now mostly a matter of historical interest. We give full credit to the Wright Brothers for inventing the airplane at about the same time Freud invented psychotherapy, but we would not today choose one of their planes if we wished to go somewhere. We have learned a lot about flying since then. Further, we can be pretty sure from what we know of their wide-ranging and forward-looking minds that, if they were alive today, Wilbur and Orville would prefer to cross the country in a 747 rather than in one of their primitive aircraft, and Freud, if he were alive today, would choose a much more modern form of psychotherapy for himself or a patient.

Nevertheless, Freud's basic ideas have been incorporated in much of the modern work and methods. Freud was a physician before he was a psychiatrist, and when he first designed psychotherapy, he built into it the basic structure of medical practice. This consists of three questions the physician asks himself or herself when a person comes into the consulting room. The first is "Why is this person here—what symptoms does he have that have brought him to my office?" The second is, "What is the hidden cause of these symptoms

—the bacterial infection, the lesion, the cyst, the vitamin deficiency, etc." The third is, "What can we do about it?" When a person comes into a psychotherapist's office, the same questions apply: "What is wrong—what are the symptoms that bring this person to my office? What is the hidden cause? What can we do about it?"

These three questions form a *method* for dealing with problems that has been built so firmly into the basic "bone structure" of psychotherapy it is hard to conceive of a therapy built on any other foundation. The method has often served us well in alleviating human suffering and pain. Applying it to the field of psychotherapy was one of Freud's great epoch-making ideas. For some problems it is absolutely necessary to use this route. Very often real change can be accomplished in this way. It is not easy, real change never is, but it can often be done if you have dedication and courage. However, in the modern approach, particularly in what we call "wholistic medicine" (see Chapter 8 for a fuller description of this) we have a second option. It is this second method that I have been particularly suggesting in this book. This approach is not based on the three questions of classic psychotherapy and of medicine generally. It is an approach to change that is based on two other questions. These are: "What is the special lifestyle, the special ways of being, relating, creating that are 'right' for this person, that will make this person glad to get up in the morning, that will give him a zest and enthusiasm for life so that when he is tired it will be mostly the 'good tired,' not the 'dragged out tired'?" And the second question is, "How can we move in that direction? Given the realities of the situation, how can we upgrade this person's life so that it becomes more like what he really wants, what he was built for?"

Using this method, a person attempts to change his total ecology by changing his life in positive directions even if he does not feel or believe that he "deserves" a better life. On page 52 I wrote about Pascal's statement about what to do if you have lost your faith. Here we are applying this idea in another sphere—we are saying that if you treat yourself as if you are worth treating well, the knowledge and the belief that this is so are likely to follow. We cannot take control of our feelings, nor are we responsible for them. We can, however, take control of our actions and assume responsibility for how we treat ourselves. When we use this approach, we look at our life and make a conscious decision to upgrade it.

AT FIRST GLANCE this might seem to be a selfish and narcissistic way to approach our life. It reminds us of what used to be called the "me-too generation" in the 1970s. However, the opposite is actually true. As we look more and more deeply into our inner life, into what we really want, we find that we, as a species, are social beings, and that we need and want good relationships with others. The healthier we are, the closer we are to our real being, the more we find that this includes good relationships in which we express and receive positive feelings. Whether we explain this on the basis of a long infantile period of dependency during which we learn to need the caring of others, or if we explain it on a basis of a gregarious instinct, or on any other basis, we find that we only attain real humanness, real joy, and real zest in our life through good and loving relationships with other human beings. When we cannot achieve this type of relationship, we often try other routes, such as making people fear us or give us tokens in the form of medals or testimonials. As the Macbeths found out, however, these other routes generally turn out to be far from satisfactory. Nicolae Ceauşescu, the dictator of Romania, and his wife Elena, demanded that in return for a certain trade agreement, the British government arrange to have them made Fellows of the Royal Society, an honor that is given only for outstanding scientific accomplishments. The British government refused, but even if it had acceded to the demand, it is highly unlikely that the satisfaction of receiving an honor they clearly did not earn would have given the Ceaușescus more than momentary satisfaction.

⌇

ONE ASPECT OF the entire concept of wholistic health is that a human being, to be considered "healthy," must demonstrate, by actual work, that he is concerned with more than himself and his own family. He must do something to show that he is related to a larger segment of the human race than just those who live in his house. The important point about this, however, is that we *first* explore ourselves and find out who we are, and then we see how this "self" needs to express itself in terms of the larger whole. We do not first take care of others in order to find or protect the self; rather, we first look within and in discovering who we are, we find that we are a social being who needs good relationships with others to express ourselves and to grow. I have former patients who work one or two evenings a week for peace groups, ecology groups, the Big Brothers or Big Sisters, as literacy volunteers, or what have you. But each of these people first looked within for what he needed to express in order to have access to more of himself, and then took up these activities for healthily selfish reasons!

⌇

SO, WITH THE understanding that I am not talking about, a "for me and against them" approach, let us get back to the method I have been describing of changing one's total ecology by changing one's life in positive directions. This is fine talk, but what does it actually mean in reality? How can we make it concrete and specific for each of us?

⁀

IN ORDER TO attempt to answer these last questions, let us try some paper and pencil exercises. (Those presented here are from a list of fifty or so in a book of mine called *Cancer as a Turning Point*,* in which I try to teach people with cancer to so change their total ecology that their inner healing ability will be brought more strongly to the aid of the medical program.) It is better and more effective if these exercises are actually done with paper and pencil rather than just in your mind. They seem to have a greater tendency to help you change. Take your time with them. These are not "quickies," but demand a good deal of thought if they are to have an effect. I strongly suggest that you do only one a day. And be warned: these are not simple. They have *Teeth* in them, and one or another may bite you. Buy or find a small notebook for this, or, if you regularly keep a private journal, write the exercises in that.

## EXERCISE #1

### PART A

You look at your schedule and you decide that there is one afternoon (or full day or evening) that you can take *just for yourself*. During this time, everyone else is on their own, it is just for you. (You may have to make some arrangements in advance like hiring a baby-sitter or telling others in the family where the

---

* *New York: Dutton, 1989; New York: Penguin-Plume, 1994.*

nearest fast-food place is, or how to buy and cook a TV dinner!) This time is for you alone and should not be used for resting so that you can be efficient the rest of the week or for doing your laundry! It is a gift of time you give yourself, and you use the time as if it were chosen by a friend who knew you as well as you do and who loved you without qualifications.

What would you do in these special "gift" periods? What activity would you choose that would give the most added richness to your life? Think of this as a special opportunity to increase your enjoyment of and participation in your own life. Describe how you would use this time.

## PART B

Do you think you will really take this time for yourself? Very few of us have a schedule so tight and demanding that we could not do this. (You might sometimes find it easier if you make a trade with someone else in the family. He or she takes off one afternoon or a full day or evening and you take off another.) If you are not going to take off this time, what is it in you that keeps you from doing it? If you are going to, what has kept you from giving yourself this gift in the past?

## *EXERCISE #2*

## PART A

Each of us engages in, or has engaged in, activities that make us feel younger and more vital. During the time we are doing them we tend to have periods when we forget everything else. Then we may suddenly look up and see that time has passed; maybe we even skipped lunch and never noticed. Afterward, we are sort of charged up; we feel good and maybe a bit tired, but it is the "good" kind of feeling tired, not the "dragged-out" kind.

When I first listed for myself those activities that fit into this class, I found that they included walking on beaches, going to "Star Wars" and James Bond movies, working in a research library, seeing operas by Puccini, learning a new field of knowledge, writing a book, giving seminars.

List the activities that turn *you* on in this way. Think back as well as in the present. Take your time.

## Part B

Just as there are activities that make you feel *more* alive and vital, there are those that tend to have the opposite effect. After engaging in these we often feel the "dragged out" kind of tired. These are activities we would prefer not to do, but in which we engage for other reasons. When I first listed for myself those that fit into this class, they included shopping for clothes, answering mail, going to dinners or parties where there are more than six other people, going to restaurants where there is loud music.

Activities may move from one list to the other as you develop. For example, two activities that for me belonged at one time on the "more alive" list and are now on the "less alive" list are reading science fiction and working full time as a psychotherapist.

List all those activities that make you feel *less*

vital and alive. Think back as well as in the present. Take your time.

## Part C

In the most recent period of your life (you define this term), how much of a conscious and at least partially successful effort have you made to so shape your life that you experience more of the "more alive" activities and fewer of the "less alive" ones?

There is an old bit of wisdom which says: "Don't worry about what the world wants from you. Worry about what makes you more alive because what the world *needs* are people who are more alive."

Describe the efforts you have made in the most recent period to change your life in this direction.

## Part D

What *in you* makes it hard to do this—to reshape your life in this way? Try, in your answer, not to blame others. For example, do not say things like, "My husband/wife wants this or that of me." Say rather something such as, "When I think my husband/wife wants this or that of me, I feel very guilty if I do not do it. It is *my* guilt feelings that make me . . ." Or "It is my anxiety when I do not feel that I measure up to what others appear to expect of me." Try to be very honest with yourself. What in you makes it hardest to "upgrade" your life so that you spend more time in activities on your "A" list and less time in activities on your "B" list?

## EXERCISE #3

**PART A**

There is an old saying: "On the day before you die, get your house in order." Since, except in very rare circumstances (very few of us are sentenced to be executed on a specific date!), we do not know in advance on what day we will die, this clearly means that we should get our house in order *today*.

After careful thought, what does it mean to you to do this? Clearly it refers to relationships with others and with yourself, and perhaps for some of us with the universe at large, rather than to dusting the furniture or mowing the lawn. Write what you would have to do *today* if you followed this advice.

**PART B**

In Part A of this exercise, you described those things you would have to do to fix up your life—to "get your house in order." What in you has kept you from doing these things in the past? Is this the same thing that makes it so hard to do them now?

**PART C**

Do you think that you will do these things in the next period of your life? If not, what would have to happen for you to do them?

## EXERCISE #4

### PART A

Suppose that a strange magical event happened to-night and when you woke up you found that your worst and most troublesome inner problem had vanished, had been cured while you slept. I am not talking about the kind of problem that is dependent on what others do or on external circumstances beyond your control, but the kind of problem that concerns how you react and wish that you didn't. Take a few moments, or as long as you need, to get clear on what specific problem this is for you.

(Remember that you are the world's outstanding expert on how you feel. If anyone can define this problem, it is you.)

Now that you have defined this problem that vanishes during the night, when you wake up, how would you know it was gone? What would you observe in your own feelings and/or behavior that would make you realize it was no longer with you? Write in detail the description of what you would observe tomorrow.

### PART B

Now that you are clear about this problem, now that you are clear about how you are with it and how you would be without it, exactly how helpless are you in regard to it?

What have you tried to do about it? Some of your efforts probably fell in the "techniques and gimmicks" class, such as counting ten before you say anything when you are unreasonably angry or taking a hard workout in the gym when your unwanted feelings rise above a certain level. These approaches are frequently helpful, but as I pointed out earlier, they rarely change anything in the long term. Or you may have tried the route of analyzing your reactions, where in your past the strength of this reaction came from and what is the unconscious meaning of the stimuli that provoke it. Clearly this was not successful since you listed it as the chief inner problem you have now.

Would the second route, that of so changing your inner ecology that your energies are directed in new ways—ways that fulfill you and give you zest and enthusiasm for your life and no longer flow in the old and troublesome paths—solve the problem? Perhaps the answer to this question is yes, and this may be the method you will have to use if you wish to end this problem. Perhaps it is time for you to take active steps to so upgrade your life that this problem vanishes in the general change.

Describe on paper exactly what you have done about this problem. What more might you have done? What in you makes it so hard to take active steps to deal with it better? What do you think you will do about it in the near future?

### EXERCISE #5

The meditation I am about to describe is based on a story told by Fyodor Dostoyevsky. (Freud was once asked who he thought were the three greatest psy-

chologists who ever lived. He replied that Dostoyevsky was clearly the first, Goethe the second. As for
the third, said Freud, "Modesty forbids!")

The story concerns a man named Ivan who lived
in Moscow and was married and had a successful
business. One day in middle life, he began to be
haunted by a devil. The devil had hooves and horns
and all the usual appurtenances, but no one could
see or hear him except Ivan. The devil kept whispering in Ivan's ear to be suspicious of everyone around
him. It said things such as, "Don't trust this man."
"Watch out for that one, he is going to cheat you."
"Don't believe this person, he hates you," and so
forth. The angrier Ivan grew at the devil, the larger it
became and the louder its voice sounded in his ear.
As Ivan became more and more suspicious of others,
and less and less trusting, his relationships became
worse and worse. Presently his wife took the children and left him and his business became less and
less profitable.

Finally his business was about to go into bank-
ruptcy and there was only one last chance to recoup
and start it up again. The chance would come at a
meeting with some of his old customers. Ivan went
downtown to the office determined that for once he
was going to react to these people with the trust they
deserved after long years of friendship and working
together. He swore to himself that this time he
would not succumb to suspicion and paranoia.
However, the devil followed him, constantly whispering in his ear, and he found himself so suspicious
of his old customers and their motives that he de-
stroyed his last chance of saving his business. They
left in anger and he was finally ruined.

Ivan returned home in absolute despair, thinking of suicide as the only way out. The devil followed close behind. As they came to the door of his house, Ivan had a sudden thought. He turned and invited the devil in for tea! The devil looked surprised, but agreed. Ivan told the serving girl to lay places for two at the table. She, seeing him alone, thought that he had gone crazy, but did as he ordered. Ivan served the devil tea and talked with him as one person to another. The devil began to grow more transparent and his voice got weaker and weaker.

Ivan, of course was not finished with the devil—it would be with him for a long time yet. But he had learned a new way to respond to it and lessen its control over him. With further use of this method, he might well be able to establish enough control that, devil or no, he could lead a normal life.

Dostoyevsky did not believe that people were haunted by a devil with a pitchfork and a strong smell of brimstone. He was of course speaking of the inner devil, the repetitive and unrealistic reactions within ourselves that make our life so much more difficult.

And now let us turn this story into a meditation! In the last exercise, you defined your worst and most troubling inner problem, the repetitive reaction that makes your life most difficult and painful. Work out a way to picture it; to symbolize it as an animal, a being, or an entity who whispers its message in your ear. (One man defined his worst inner problem as a tendency, when facing opposition, to react as if he were helpless and to ask his opponent for help instead of confronting the situation. It reminded him of a little dog he once had. When it had done something wrong and was being scolded, the dog would act as if it had hurt a paw and would hold up the paw as if it were in pain and whimper. He pictured his worst inner problem as that small dog and named it Sore Paws.) How would you picture yours? What would you name it?

Take your time on this. It probably needs some thought. Get the best image you can for the problem and give it the most appropriate name you can think of. It is important not to hurry at this point. You have already done something about this problem simply by defining it. Look over what you wrote in the last exercise. Think some more about it and about how to symbolize and name it.

Now get yourself comfortable. Imagine yourself in a situation that generally leads to the kind of response you have called Inner Problem Number One. Imagine the situation clearly. Now picture the image of the problem you have devised and picture it whispering its message in your ear. It is telling you to feel and behave in exactly the way you do not want to any longer.

Observe it in your imagination, perched on your shoulder or standing close to you, whispering how you should feel and behave. Listen to it and watch it. Do this as clearly as you can for three minutes the first time, five minutes the next.

Add this exercise to your meditation program. By now you are experienced enough so that you can decide how long each session with this particular meditation should be and how often would be best for you to do it.

Then, the next time you are in the kind of situation that arouses this response, try, if only for a moment, to picture the image you designed. Smile at it. Say, in effect, "Here you are again, old friend. Can you skip this particular incident? Go to the bathroom or something, I'm busy now." And so forth. Try to smile wryly at it for a second or two if you can. This may not work too effectively the first time or two. Old habits die hard and old reaction programs are resistant to change. Sometimes you may forget and other times you may be overwhelmed by the long-standing conditioning you have to react in a particular way. However, as Ivan found out, each time you try, you will gain more control and will be more likely to succeed the next time.

IN ALL THESE exercises and meditations you are, as you will probably have realized by now, taking more control of your own life and destiny. You are shaping your life closer to your heart's desire. You are also changing your inner ecology so that, after you have successfully dealt with your weight problem, the same inner forces will not operate in the same old way to reactivate it.

This reshaping can, of course, be done with or without exercises of the sort I have listed here. One can look at oneself and ask, "In the total being that I am, physical, mental, emotional, spiritual, what part of me has been most neglected? What part of me has been standing outside the door of my concern whimpering, "Is there nothing for me?" Then determine to upgrade that part of oneself. Or, to put it in more poetic (flowery?) language, you might ask yourself, "In the garden that is me, what part has received the least watering and care? How can I remedy this defect?" After taking action and upgrading one particular aspect of your being, you ask the question again and the next part that has been the most neglected is then given special care. And so forth, until you are so busy and enthusiastic living your own specific life that you no longer feel the need of improvement in this period of your lifetime.

This can be done by will and by acting as if you really cared about yourself. The action, as I have discussed before, is likely to increase the actual feeling, but it often must first be done by will power.

⌐

OFTEN, IF WE are overweight (or underweight), the problem crept up on us slowly and we were not very much aware of it until it was overwhelming. Then, it seemed to us that the focus of the problem was to readjust our weight. This is often a necessary first step, but we must redefine the problem if we wish to solve it permanently. The redefined problem is not being thin, but how to get the most zest, enthusiasm, and real enjoyment out of life. Losing weight is not an end in itself, but a necessary part of the road to this enhancement of positive feeling.

When a person's weight is not at a healthy level for him, it is the person's total life that must ultimately be treated. Being over- or underweight is a sign that there is something wrong, and what is wrong is not just a weight problem. It may be a glandular problem, and then that is what must be dealt with. It may, more likely today, be a problem of the relationship the person has with himself, with others, and/or with the universe at large. (For example, the problem of determining the meaning of one's life and existence, whether one's efforts have a real purpose and, if so, what that is, is much more widespread than is generally realized, and it often has serious effects on all the person's systems of action and reaction. The psychiatrist Carl Jung once remarked that he had never seen a patient over thirty-five years of age whose problem was not at bottom a religious one and whose psychological problems were not cured when his religious problem was successfully dealt with. Jung was not, of course, speaking about problems of church attendance and church dogma. He was speaking rather about problems related to the meaning and purpose in life.)

Storing fat is a natural body function. The body burns fat all day and this burning accounts for more than half the energy you expend in your daily life. What has gone wrong is not that you eat too much or exercise too little, but that the balance has gone out of the eating-energy-storage system. We have all seen people who ate a great deal, exercised very little, and still remained slim. And, by and large, overweight people do not eat more than people whose weight is normal for them. Carefully controlled studies have shown that on the exact same diet some people will remain at the same weight, some will lose, and some will gain. It is a matter of your total organization of body, mind, and spirit.

With some conditions involving a variation from the norm it is necessary to treat the symptom before you can treat the central cause. We see this in depression, which is an extremely painful condition whose chief symptom is feeling terrible about oneself and the world in general. One cannot treat the cause until one has treated the symptom. Today, depressive feelings are treated with antidepressive drugs and then the underlying causes are amenable to psychotherapy. Psychotherapy for the real problem is generally not possible until the symptom has been treated.

With weight problems it is usually necessary to treat the symptom first and to attain a healthy body weight. Then the underlying problems that made us lose control of our eating-energy-storage system become more amenable to treatment. Unless we deal with the underlying problems, however, the weight problem is likely to recur as soon as we go off our diet, just as, in the case of depression, the depressive feelings will recur as soon as we go off the drugs.

# ·8·

≈

# The Meaning of Wholistic Health

·

That any sane nation, having observed that you could provide for the supply of bread by giving bakers a pecuniary interest in baking for you, should go on to give surgeons a pecuniary interest in cutting off your leg, is enough to make one despair of political humanity.

—George Bernard Shaw

*W*E ARE BOMBARDED by the media with the message that "your health is a mess. To stave off disaster, you should immediately take a medication or see a professional." Lewis Thomas, president of New York's Memorial Sloan-Kettering Cancer Center, wrote:

*Nothing has changed so much in the past twenty-five years as the public's perception of its own health. The change amounts to a loss of confidence in the human form. The general belief these days seems to be that the body is fundamentally flawed, subject to disintegration at any moment, always on the verge of mortal disease, always in need of continual monitoring and support by health-care professionals.*

Our new view is close to that of many primitive societies, that death is unnatural; that it should not happen. The primitive says that a witch or a demon caused it. The modern says that the doctor failed to prevent it.

There is a tremendous amount of propaganda from drug

companies and their advertising agencies designed to convince us that our bodies do not work and are constantly in danger of decomposing from one thing or another. We must, we are warned, keep a large variety of drugs available, or we will certainly be overcome by everything from dandruff to hemorrhoids and athlete's foot. Not a single system of the body (excluding those like the lymphatic system, which the lay public does not really believe exist) is exempted from the threat that it cannot function well by itself or recover unaided if it becomes disordered. We are further warned that there are really severe and terrible problems awaiting us and that we had better prepare for them by giving money to specialized foundations so that their research can be further advanced by the time we or someone close to us is felled by their particular dread disease. There is no effective counter-propaganda around. No agency exists for the celebration of the fact that most people are, in real life, free of active disease and will recover from any minor indisposition by themselves. No one takes public note of the truth of the matter, which is that most people in this country have a clear, unimpeded run at a longer lifetime than could have been foreseen by an earlier generation.

Indeed one of the easiest ways to make people angry at you (try it on your friends and watch them become your former friends) is to tell them that they do *not* need more medical care, vitamins, exercise, dietary expertise, or constant concern about their health. This kind of suggestion has become the equivalent of a personal attack in most circles and will generally elicit the same response you would get if you were to light a cigarette in a health food store.

In spite of the fact that the amount of money spent in this country on medical care rose from $10 billion in 1950 to $250 billion in 1980, we all feel that the medical system is underfinanced and inadequate, that physicians are too hurried and overworked, and that there are not enough nurses. Further, if you examine medical progress, there should logically have been a lowering of health costs. A typical case of lobar pneumonia, preantibiotic, involved three or four weeks of hospitalization; typhoid was a twelve to sixteen-week illness; meningitis often required several months of care through convalescence; these and other common infectious diseases can now be aborted promptly, within just a few days. The net result of the anti-infection technology ought to have been a very large decrease in the cost of care.

We feel angry when we are told that our pumping more money into the medical system has long since reached a point of diminishing returns; that we are, as a nation, remarkably free of disease—far more so than at any other period in history; that our bodies are generally capable of taking care of themselves; and that we should stop feeling guilty about not taking better care of our physical being. Hearing these things, we feel as if we were being attacked and something were being taken away from us.

And, indeed, something is being taken away. It is the hope of magic: the hope that medicine (with its magicians dressed in white coats) will solve all our problems; postpone death until we are ready—or, perhaps, forever—and make us "healthy," and full of zest, joy, and sexual attractiveness and ability. Anyone who takes away the hope that we can achieve heaven on earth simply by taking a few more milligrams of vitamin C *plus* zinc *plus* vitamin E each day is going to be cordially disliked. Our belief in the magical promise of medicine is an illusion of our entire culture today, and anyone who tries to remove that belief does so at his peril.

However, there is a reason to try to give up this illusion, and to point out its fallacy. The illusion leads to a blocking of our perceptions, so that we cannot see how we can validly work toward our own health. It leads to the placement of tremendous and unfair loads on the medical profession, and to a continuing and increasing hostility between the physician and the lay public as medical capabilities do not live up to the impossible hopes we have for them. It is also turning us into a nation of angry and overmedicated hypochondriacs.

Paradoxically, we are, as a culture, extremely discontented with the entire medical system. An HEW study reported that only 7 percent of Americans identified themselves as "feeling good most of the time." How did we get into this predicament?

There are, I believe, three major ways to account for it:

1. The rise of the mechanical view in Western society and the concomitant idea that *everything* can be fixed and made to run perfectly.

2. The tremendous advances of medicine in the last half of this century in control of the communicable and infectious diseases led to the idea that *all* diseases could be controlled.

3. The confusion that identified health as "an absence of disease." This semantic disaster led us to the idea we would be "healthy" when free of disease.

Since we all knew we wanted something called "health" very badly, but had not defined it, and since we knew that it was something we could get by curing "sickness," an entire industry grew up to try to satisfy this need. Working on the principle that if what you are doing doesn't work, the answer is to do it more—if the bolt does not fit the nut, force it until it does—medical procedures became more and more extensive. The use of surgery, drugs, yearly medical examinations, tonics, vitamins, and so forth increased exponentially. As with any competitive industry, the means often replaced the end, and what could be sold became as much a hallmark of validity as did the products' effectiveness. Many of the procedures and products were useless (such as yearly examinations and wholesale tonsil removal) and some were downright dangerous (the thalidomide and DES disasters are examples).

A part of our present problem is a linguistic one. We tend to speak of a disease as a "thing," and not as part of a total life process. We thereby separate the person and the illness. This automatically leads us back to the old demon theory of disease in which a demon was believed to have invaded the body and had to be dispossessed. As soon as the demon was driven out, the person was cured. It would be far more realistic, in terms of modern knowledge (and would improve our ability to solve problems in this area), to restructure our language so that when we spoke or thought about illness, the language would indicate that the specific individual had tensions, strengths, and weaknesses in his relationship with himself, others, and the cosmos, and that this total gestalt was showing symptoms of carcinoma or of angina pectoris. We would then automatically see any healing process as having two interrelated parts: emergency treatment of the symptom and long-term reorganization of the total pattern of the person's life.

Because we see the disease and the illness as a "thing" that has happened to us, we seek a single "cause." The use of "fate" or "happenstance" to explain untoward events is no more acceptable in our society than is the evil eye of a bad-tempered witch doctor. We may, for example, lay the blame on "carcinogens" in the air, forgetting that while these are a real threat to our defense systems, they do not affect all persons equally exposed in the same way. Nevertheless, it is useful and soothing to have an acceptable demon out there and to attempt—as we should and must—to clean up our air and water. It is important that we do this, but if we believe that these outside factors are the sole cause of illness, we are going to be disappointed and depressed if we eventually do have air that is fit for us and our children to breathe and disease continues. The environment is only one factor in the pattern, not the sole "cause" of illness.

We often try to blame other people—"My boss caused the heart attack by being such a bastard"—although, unless we have a sizable paranoid streak in our personality makeup, this kind of explanation doesn't feel very satisfying for very long. Since Freud, a new explanation has become popular in our culture. In our society psychosomatic explanations of illness have become extremely popular because they allow patients to fix the blame on the most comforting locus of all —themselves. The idea that there is a single cause for illness, that something or someone must be to blame, can often be heard in the sound of a patient's voice as he asks his physician: "Why have I contracted this disease?" The tone implies that something underhanded is going on. We want there to be a simple cause, preferably something outside ourselves, and to know that we contracted the disease by chance. The answer, "A virus," and the assurance that "There's a lot of it going around," fits our wishes exactly. We can neglect to ask why others similarly exposed did not also contract the disease. We want the doctor to be able to repel the invader with no particular inconvenience to ourselves (except perhaps for a shot, a pill, and a few days in bed) and with no implication that the illness may be telling us something about taking on further responsibility for our own lives.

The idea of one specific cause for each disease, and therefore, one specific cure, fits in well with another of our fantasies.

There is a very old belief among human beings that somewhere there exists a "natural" remedy, a plant or an herb, that will solve all human medical problems and give us health and youth forever—in short, that will make us immortal. This belief goes back at least to Sumerian times. We find it in the Gilgamesh saga probably composed before 3000 B.C. The surgeon and philosopher Kenneth Walker thinks that this belief comes in part from our observations of the behavior of animals, which will often treat themselves for wounds or illness by eating certain plants or by using certain materials in their natural environment. Birds, for example, are very successful at ridding themselves of insect parasites by means of dust baths. (It is only recently that we have understood that this works by clogging up the respiratory pores of the insects.) The belief is very persistent, and finds its modern equivalent in many of the kooky fad diets and advertisements for over-the-counter remedies that clutter up the media. So deeply ingrained is this idea in Western culture that one nineteenth-century German medical research scientist, Brown-Sequard, felt it necessary to try to disabuse his students and associates of it by putting a plaque over the entrance to his laboratory: *"Gegen den Tod ist keine Kraut gewachsen"* (Against death no herbs do grow).

The widespread fantasy of a golden age that preceded our own (whatever our own might be) has also strengthened the present concept of sickness and health. We have a feeling that in a previous age human beings were happier and healthier than they are now. If we stop to think about it, we quickly realize that this is not so, but the notion persists and influences our viewpoint to a very marked degree. We feel, for example, that in the small town of sixty years ago (a sort of cross between Andy Hardy's hometown and a stage set for Thornton Wilder's *Our Town*) with its good and caring physician (probably looking a bit like Lionel Barrymore) there was less sickness. Thus, the nutritionists blame most of today's illness on chemical additives in our food, and the American Cancer Society blames most cancers on environmental carcinogens produced by the industry of our time. Both of these theories seem reasonable until we look at the mortality statistics of the past century and it becomes clear that these explanations are too simplistic.

As one example, I might mention that in Egyptian mummies (from the best families of Egypt, long before environmental poisons and food additives, and when tobacco was unknown), we find ample evidence of widespread tumors, arthritis, caries, silicosis, pneumonia, pleurisy, rheumatism, kidney stones, cirrhosis of the liver, mastoiditis, appendicitis, meningitis, smallpox, TB, and a wide variety of other conditions.

The idea of a golden age of health preceding our own is not new. In 1796, the physician C. W. Hufeland wrote that mankind was on the road to physical degeneration and a higher early death rate, unless it returned to the simple ways of life of the good old times "in ways agreeable to nature."

Since Rousseau in particular, and the French Revolution in general, we have subscribed to the widely held idea that society causes illnesses, and that in a "natural state" (whatever that means) or in a "good society" (defined by the beliefs of the moment), people would be healthy and not fall prey to disease. (The latest version of this notion is the rapidly growing belief that *everything* produced by modern technology is carcinogenic.) Further to this idea is the belief that once the revolution (the changes *we* advocate) is complete, people will be free of disease. The excuses offered when this does not happen are as ingenious and plentiful among revolutionists as they are among Christian Scientists.

It must be made clear that what I am saying here is not intended as a criticism of physicians, but rather as an analysis of the present-day structure of medicine and its position in our society. The physician is generally in practice for serious and positive motives, and is under more pressure from the status and structure of his profession than is the layman.

In the 1940s, the World Health Organization defined health as "a state of complete physical, mental, and social well-being." This definition places a tremendous burden on those who are expected to deal with health problems: the members of the medical profession. They are rather well equipped to deal with the first third of the definition (physical), ill equipped to deal with the second (mental), and completely unequipped to deal with the third (social). Neither were they trained to deal with the constant interaction among the three, nor to recognize that the definition omits a crucial part of what it means to be human—the spiritual, the deep and basic need to have a meaningful framework for existence. Forgotten was the obvious fact, shown throughout history, that human beings will often sacrifice their physical well-being in order to satisfy their spiritual needs.

It is a function of the swing of the cultural pendulum that today the welfare of a population is considered almost entirely in secular terms. In reaction to the medieval view that the welfare of the soul was of primary importance, we have, since the eighteenth century, been moving in the opposite direction, toward the view that the welfare of the body is of primary importance. This is one reason we have been concerned with "sickness" (something wrong with the entire organism). The months of meetings of the council of the French Revolution on how best to replace the clergy with a medical bureaucracy was a very clear example of this development, which we are only now beginning seriously to challenge.

As "health" came to be seen merely as the absence of "sickness," increasingly the problems associated with being human tended to be included in the definition of illness. During the past sixty years, the physician has been assigned more and more tasks—many of which he has had no training in handling. The lack of "happiness," "fulfillment," and "zest in life," has been defined as illness. This is a problem he is expected to be able to "cure." None of these, of course, are mechanical problems and so they are out of the range of the basic system around which medical training is organized.

So great has been the medicalization of American society, to use an expression of the biometrician Renee Fox, that the hospital is displacing the church or the parliament as the archetypical institution of Western society. Disapproved behavior is coming to be considered an illness requiring treatment rather than a crime requiring punishment or a sin requiring conversion.

Anything the physician is willing to deal with becomes an illness, thus reinforcing the implication that only physicians are able to deal with it or that they are more effective in dealing with the problem than anyone else. The physician says that he is willing to treat alcoholism, since it is a negative deviation from a norm and that is how he defines a disease. Alcoholism thus *becomes* a disease, and the physician's prerogative to treat, even though he does not know the cause and has no reason to suspect that it is biological. Further, there is no reason to suspect that he is more effective in dealing with it than are the courts or the church, and he is demonstrably less successful than the peer treatment of AA.

Medicalization has gone so far that we no longer even believe in our ability to die alone or in the warmth of the company of our loved ones. We feel that we must have around us a court of white-coated antiseptic figures to make the final transition. The individual has come to feel so helpless that he cannot even wrestle with his own death or find his own path to it.

Before the beginning of this century, the modern physician's caseload was shared with another class of professionals. A large part of his present practice went to the religious (or "wise") advisers of the community. Problems they once handled, and which now come to the consulting room, include: addictive disorders such as alcoholism, drug abuse, obesity, the "worried well" (who make up such a large part of the physician's everyday medical work), certain types of physical violence such as that leading to the "battered child" or "battered wife" syndrome, existential crises, inability to conceive or to stop conceiving, discontent with a job or love life, bed-wetting, sexual deviance and dysfunction, anorexia nervosa, mental or physical exhaustion, difficulty in relating to others, inability to find meaning in life, and unhappiness. Even pregnancy is—in practice—generally regarded as a nine-month self-limiting illness, often requiring surgery at the end.

In the Soviet Union under Stalin, disagreement with the dictates of the Central Committee was seen as prima facie evidence of mental illness, and the political dissident was likely to become a medical "patient" and wind up in a mental hospital. A belief that you could change or improve the social or political situation was defined as "sluggish schizophrenia" for which incarceration in a psychiatric hospital was the treatment. In Maoist China, mental illness was perceived as a political problem and Maoist politicians were placed in charge of psychotic deviants. (It is not clear if this has recently changed.) The psychotic was perceived as a person who was—at least unconsciously—a class enemy who needed criticism and self-criticism to make him politically active and therefore healthy.

In the United States we do the same thing, but generally limit the punishment to children who have no vote. Those children who object to poor teaching and poor educational theory are turned over to the medical arm of the establishment for drugging and retraining. The belief is that drugs such as Ritalin will cure them of their objections to an educational system on the brink of disaster. (We also do occasionally use medical definitions for political purposes. Two cases in this category would be those of Ezra Pound and General James Walker.)

As for the use of drugs for "hyperactive" children (that is to say, children who aren't school-adjusted), our present approach is also used by at least one primitive culture. Among the Jivaro Indians of South America (one of the most hostile and aggressive societies ever discovered), if a child consistently misbehaves he is forcibly administered a very powerful hallucinogen (datura). The theory is that this will enable him to perceive "reality" correctly, and he will then start to behave. How this approach differs from our own (except in the choice of drug) escapes my understanding.

Further, the physician must now decide who may drive a car, stay away from work, immigrate, become a soldier; who is competent to know right from wrong, or is likely to be dangerous to himself or others, or is too hopelessly ill to be worthy of further lifesaving devices; who is too incompetent to manage his own affairs; who receives the first available organ for transplant, and who must wait. With this kind of assignment and the kind of training they get, is it any wonder that physicians have such high heart attack, drug-abuse, and suicide rates? (Suicide is the second most common cause of death for medical students and is more frequent among physicians than the combined deaths from automobile accidents, airplane crashes, homicides, and drownings. Drugs and alcohol account for at least one third of the time physicians as a group spend hospitalized during their careers.)

With the medicalization of American society, the physician now has the power to legitimize one's "illness" (the feeling of being sick) by conceding that one actually has a disease. He also has the power to deny this legitimacy. If you are not ill in the correct ways with the correct symptoms, you are labeled a hypochondriac, a malingerer (if you seem to be gaining a financial advantage), or a neurotic. The penalties for being sick in incorrect ways can range from social ostracism to denial of workmen's compensation funds. The penalties for being sick in incorrect ways in the Army or in prison are obvious.

The nineteenth-century definition of medicine, still used in medical schools today, was "The science concerned with the prevention and cure of disease." The authoritative *Stedman's Medical Dictionary* defines disease as: "Morbus, Illness, Sickness. An interuption or perversion of functions of any of the organs, a morbid change in any of the tissues or an abnormal state of the body as a whole, continuing for a longer or shorter period." This is what the physician has been trained to cope with, and essentially *all* the physician has been trained to cope with.

In every profession, a certain amount of "ethnocentrism" develops. (George Bernard Shaw wrote, "Every profession is a conspiracy against the layman.") The lawyer sacrifices the larger view of humanity for a concentration on property and torts, the cleric on sanctity, the academician on learning, the chef on eating, and the physician on illness and therapy. The population is seen from a specialized point of view, and actions are inevitably interpreted in light of this view rather than from a more universal perspective.

Trained to look for sickness, very often the physician can *see* only sickness and cannot perceive normal functioning. Individual variations in function and in behavior are much too easily perceived as pathology. In one experiment eight pseudo patients had themselves admitted to mental institutions by saying they heard voices. Thereafter they behaved normally. The entire staff remained convinced they were "schizophrenics," as they had been labeled upon admittance, and did not recognize their lack of psychosis. The staff did not seem capable of recognizing normal behavior in patients, although some of the other patients suspected the impersonations. An experiment with highly trained psychoanalysts produced much the same results.

Because of the general attitude that has developed—that health is an absence of sickness, and that the physician must take the active role and "do something" about each problem —the physician and the patient have painted themselves into a very difficult corner. The task of the physician is to "fix" the problem and the responsibility is seen as his, not the patient's. When we go to a physician with a problem, we have very much the same attitude that we have when we take our car to a mechanic. "It's slow to start in the morning," we say. "Please fix it." We expect the mechanic to do something physically, not to tell the car that it must change its attitude, its owner, or that it is an Oldsmobile and has been living its life as if it were a Buick just because Buicks are the admired cars this year. We do not expect the mechanic to tell us that the car has the ability to fix itself and that we have to find out what is blocking this ability. If he cannot fix the car, we call him an incompetent and find another mechanic who will.

When we approach a physician in the same way—and, being a creature of the same culture, the physician has the same attitudes and expectations we have—we force him to "do something" about the problem. The result is that the patient generally leaves the office medicated, frequently overmedicated, sometimes with completely unnecessary surgical procedures scheduled. And all because we regard ourselves as machines to be fixed rather than organisms to be gardened.

A gardener has quite a different attitude. If something is wrong with the development of a plant, the gardener will examine the total environment in which the plant exists and to which it is responding. How do its genetically determined needs and potentialities interact with the environment? (In human beings we call this interaction the "lifestyle.") The gardener will then determine what the plant needs—more or less sun, minerals, acid-base balance in its nourishment, space around it, and so on. (To continue the analogy to humans, which of its physical, mental, interpersonal, or spiritual needs are under, over, or wrongly fed?) The gardener deals with the whole—with the organism in an environment. The mechanic fixes nonfunctioning parts. This is why it seems plain that for human "sickness" and "health," two different attitudes are needed. Although some wise professionals may be able to encompass both, it seems clear that for the foreseeable future we are going to need two separate sets of professionals working together.

A machine is "sick" when it is not functioning efficiently and needs a mechanic to fix it. It is "healthy" when it is running smoothly and does not need a mechanic. Similarly, in spite of all the definitions and arguments, Western culture defines a human being as sick when he needs a physician and healthy when he does not. *The modern definition of health is the absence of sickness.* When you analyze all the current talk about "health care delivery systems," you find that these words simply mean systems for connecting an individual whom the culture defines as sick to a medical practitioner. In fact, there are no such things as "health care delivery systems," there are only connection systems for sick people and physicians.

That the present-day medical view of humans is the same as that of mechanics toward machines can be shown in a wide variety of examples. One would be that "underachieving" is seen as a problem to be "fixed," while "overachieving" is not. A machine needs fixing when it is not efficient enough, not when it is too efficient.

However, every gardener and every farmer knows that this is not true of living organisms. For a plant to grow beyond its optimum rate or beyond its optimum size is a sign of real trouble and breakdown. Overachievement in a plant is seen as a problem. In a machine or a human, it is not.

When a physician, viewing a patient's aging body as a rapidly wearing-out machine, says—or agrees with the patient's statement—that a symptom is due to aging, or when he says something idiotic such as, "What can you expect at your age? You know you're not a spring chicken anymore," he is reinforcing the patient's sense that he is losing control, his feelings of impotence and gradual dissolution in the face of an inexorable process. The reinforcement of his helplessness weakens the patient's ability to fight for control of his life. If you told an artist that his paintings would eventually decay and be lost, you would be telling him a truth. You certainly would not be helping the development of his creativity.

A more meaningful answer might be, "Let us see what we can do to lessen the effect of the symptom, if we cannot erase it completely, and let us go on to see in what ways the entire fabric of your life can be enhanced and made richer and more colorful." An answer of this sort reinforces the patient's sense of himself as a human being and aids him in taking control of his own destiny.

The physician will frequently say to the patient something like, "A lot depends on your attitude." What he usually means is this: "If you are a good patient and do as I say, and if you do not ask uncomfortable questions, it will be a lot easier on me and I will not have to deal with you as a human being who is suffering." One patient with a severe cancer observed that his physicians all spoke about his attitude and how important it was, but became extremely uncomfortable and changed the subject when he or his family mentioned activities such as prayer, support groups, psychic healing, meditation, or psychotherapy—all things you do to change your attitude. By and large, physicians who advocate positive attitudes are unhappy with any discussion of techniques to attain them, except the most superficial approaches. Thus Carl Simonton—who prescribes meditation for his cancer patients as well as mainstream medical techniques (he is a Board-certified radiologist)—is often dismissed by other cancer physicians because his methods go against their basic assumptions—that they are dealing with the problems of a machine and that there is something queer and upsetting in the notion of dealing with a machine's mind (or attitude). The same thing is true of the way many physicians regard their psychiatric colleagues. They feel that as soon as the psychiatrist does anything but administer drugs, he is departing from "real medicine," that he has left the province of science (which they see as the nineteenth-century mechanistic model of physics) and is trafficking in softheaded irrelevancies.

Every experienced physician knows that a deadly symptom has appeared when a patient with a serious disease says, "I just don't care about getting better. Life doesn't mean very much to me." Or other statements of this sort. Conversely, the physician also knows the importance of the will to live, and the significance of the general patterns of a person's life in determining the outcome of disease. In addition, he has seen how often premature retirement leads to decline and death, and how infants who are not held and loved enough die at a much higher rate from all causes than do infants not so deprived. However, because of the physician's mechanistic training and viewpoint, and because he basically sees himself—and is seen by his patients—as a repairman, he tends to become extremely uncomfortable in the presence of approaches that *do something* about these factors. Psychiatry is seen as inferior to "real" medicine; meditation and prayer are seen at worst as superstitions or as weak occupational therapy at best. The physician, therefore, tends to ignore the implications of such a proved and major symptom because it does not fit in with his system of thought. Physicians, as do other people, sometimes subscribe to the maxim, "If the fact disagrees with your theory, put the fact under the rug and out of sight."

One patient stated very well her feelings about the mechanical attitude of her physician. An angiogram had been prescribed. In this procedure a long, thin tube is inserted into an artery in the groin and carefully pushed up the artery until the end of it is inside the heart and the heart and the coronary arteries can be dyed and photographed. When this procedure was described to the patient, she felt—even as you and I would—some anxiety, and expressed a desire to meet and talk with the specialist who would perform the actual work. Her cardiologist said, "You don't have to know the person who does this. We are all good technicians here." The patient answered, "But I am not an automobile."

As part of the vast ferment going on in Western medicine today, there is a strong and growing recognition of the need to reexamine traditional concepts and definitions. All over America "wholistic" and "humanistic" physicians, clinics, and theories are springing up. A great many lay persons are rejecting mainstream medicine, in part or in whole, and are trying to solve illness and health problems with a wide variety of techniques ranging all the way from intelligent and carefully thought-out approaches to those based on outright kookiness. These techniques include nutrition, homeopathy, the devouring of vast amounts of vitamins, chanting, meditation, foot massage, manipulating the plates of the skull, wearing crystals, wearing of copper bracelets while sitting under pyramid-shaped structures, psychic healing, acupuncture, yoga, and many others. So angry and rejecting have some of these people become that they have forgotten the psychiatrist Jules Eisenbud's "First Theorem": "Just because an idea has been rejected by modern science does not mean that ipso facto it is valid."

The ancient Greek historian Herodotus described an experiment that had been done in a Persian city he visited. For one year, the authorities kept track of all patients treated by physicians and how they responded to the accepted medical techniques. Then they exiled the physicians for the following year and built a shaded portico in the center of town. All those who were sick would come there every day or have their relatives carry them there. Passersby were encouraged to talk with a sick person about his symptoms and to discuss their own ideas on the subject. The experiences of others they had known with the same symptoms would be recounted, along with the remedies that had been undertaken. The patients were free to follow any advice they wished. At the end of the year the city authorities compared the results of the two test periods (this was probably the first "controlled" medical experiment in recorded history) and decided to make the exile of the physicians permanent!

In their anger and disillusionment with modern medicine, many people would likely feel that the ancient Persians had a worthwhile idea. However, anyone who looks at the comparative mortality rates in the Persian empire (or any society before our present one) and in the modern era, would quickly see the fallacy of this concept.

The revolution in Western medicine has gone much farther than is generally realized. Physicians and nurses are studying and practicing psychic healing. Prestigious medical journals are printing articles on how to laugh your way to health, and Walter Reed Army Medical Center is holding intensive seminars on wholistic and humanistic approaches in medicine. Even the most conservative bastions of traditional medicine are questioning their own assumptions and experimenting with change.

In order to understand what is going on in medicine today, it is necessary to examine a basic conflict that has been waged continually for at least 2,500 years. This is the problem of what the physician primarily should try to do. Should he actively and forcefully *intervene* when the patient is ill by the use of surgery and strong medicaments to *conquer* the disease? Or should he instead concentrate on finding ways to support the patient's natural healing processes? In effect, should he be primarily a *mechanic* and repair the ill body, or should he be primarily a *gardener* and help the body grow past disease and toward health?

It would be foolish to argue that the physician should be completely one or the other. Both roles are clearly necessary. The most mechanically oriented surgeon is aware that the best sutures in the world can only bring the sides of the wound together in such a way that healing can take place and the patient's self-recuperative abilities can seal it. The most fervid "natural healing" devotee would agree that if an artery is cut and spouting blood, a surgical intervention is needed immediately.

Medicine is not and never has been a matter of one extreme or another. The question of emphasis, however, is extremely important and the front lines of the battle have surged back and forth since at least the time of Hippocrates. Indeed, his is the first clear statement espousing one side or the other that we have on record. He saw disease as being made up of two elements—suffering (*Pathos*) and restitutive healing attempts of the body (*Ponos*)—and believed the physician should primarily search for, try to understand, and aid the *Ponos*. Reporting this, the twelfth-century physician Maimonides wrote:

*Galen has already explained to us that the ancient Greeks, when in doubt as to what to do in a certain disease, did nothing but left the patient to Nature, which they considered sufficient to cure all illnesses. . . . And it is true that the physician should help Nature, support it and do nothing else but follow it.*

In Roman times, the conflict between those who believed in the healing powers of the body and in cooperating with them (the Hippocratics), and those who believed that this passive approach was useless, a mere "meditation on death," and that active intervention was necessary (the followers of Asclepiades of Bithynia), continued, with violent argument and vituperation on both sides.

The idea that much of what is perceived as "illness" results from the body's restorative and self-healing activities was not lost after the Classical period, but also was typical of the medieval approach. Thus, according to the Theory of Humors (the accepted medical theory of the period), it was believed that illness resulted from an excess of one of the four kinds of fluid in the body and that, when this condition occurred, certain self-healing dispositions of the body automatically went into action. For example, these dispositions raised the body temperature so as to "cook" the excess of raw fluid and then separate the cooked from the uncooked parts. The physician *cooperated* with these self-restorative dispositions. He gave warming drinks and warmed the patient externally to help with the cooking. He then helped the body to dispose of the cooked excess by administering purges and emetics and by bleeding. Thus, from the physician's viewpoint, every disease was a process he could help to regulate by cooperating with the self-healing abilities of the patient.

According to the sixteenth-century physician Paracelsus, "Man is his own doctor and finds healing herbs in his own garden. The physician is in ourselves, and in our own nature are all the things we need."

At that time, medicine was divided between the "Galenic" physicians, such as Paracelsus himself, who favored herbal preparations intended to cooperate with the body's healing efforts, and the "spagyric" physicians, who favored the use of surgery, cautery, and chemical preparations intended to intervene actively in the process of the disease. The comments they made about each other were very similar to the comments made by the opponents of "wholistic" and "mainstream" medicine today.

Once the Church permitted human dissection for medical purposes in the seventeenth century, it reinforced the idea, already developing in the philosophy of the period, that body and mind were separate and should be considered separately. The basis for the Cartesian dualism of our time was greatly strengthened. The physical body could be dissected and investigated by anatomists; the soul and mind remained the province of theology and philosophy. Since the body and the mind had been separated by the Church, and since the science of the time was mechanical, the belief took hold that the body itself was a machine, disease a consequence of the breakdown of this machine, and the physician's task was mechanical repair of the parts.

Medicine increasingly adopted the view that the physician's task was actively to intervene in and conquer disease. Gradually the idea that the body had self-healing abilities was lost. Some physicians tried to restore the older viewpoint or to strike a balance, but they were unsuccessful.

Throughout Europe and America in the eighteenth century, medical opinion was primarily on the side of active intervention against disease. The physician saw himself as the enemy of the disease process and his task to take arms against it. However, his knowledge and tools were as scant and ineffective as ever, and neither he nor those who espoused the "natural" healing methods were able to do much good. Neither school knew very much and, what was worse, most of what they were sure they knew was wrong. Both killed people by the hundreds of thousands. The "naturopaths" probably obeyed to a much greater degree Hippocrates's "First Law" (*Primum non nocere:* Above all, do no harm) because they acted less aggressively and their remedies were weaker. It may be that this is the reason why, in the early 1800s, public opinion began to favor their approach.

On one side was the Popular Health Movment (PHM) and on the other the orthodox physicians. The PHM used mostly plant and herb remedies and attacked mainstream physicians for their "barbaric" treatments, their fees, and their "arrogance." They sought to "return medicine to the people," to "make every man his own doctor," partly through Samuel Thompson's Friendly Botanical Societies. Opposing them were many leading physicians such as the French F. J. V. Broussais, who believed only active measures could cure disease because the body had no natural healing power. In the event, the PHM and its allies were so successful that in the United States, state after state repealed its laws licensing physicians, and by 1849 only New Jersey and the District of Columbia had such laws still on the books. Anyone could hang up a shingle as John Jones, Physician, or Mary Jones, Physician. It would seem that the "intervene and conquer" approach to medicine was in full rout.

Many orthodox physicians of the period also believed there should be a broader approach to the healing arts than mainstream medicine could provide. Benjamin Rush, who was Surgeon General of the Continental Army (and a signer of the Declaration of Independence), wrote:

*The Constitution of this Republic should make special*
*provision for Medical Freedom as well as Religious Free-*
*dom. . . . To restrict the art of healing to one class of*
*men and deny equal privileges to others will constitute*
*the Bastille of medical science. All such laws are un-*
*American and despotic.*

During the course of the next half century, however, the
picture was completely reversed. With two major advances
in medicine, the physicians' ability to successfully intervene
against and cure disease became greater than at any other
time in history. Germ theory and the consequent introduction of antiseptic surgery on the one hand, and medicine's
alliance with the new science of chemistry on the other, led
to a dramatic new control of many theretofore deadly diseases. Communicable and infectious diseases such as tuberculosis, smallpox, and typhus were largely brought under
control. The Sanitary Revolution of the late 1800s, when the
water supply was improved, housing laws were passed, linen
underclothing became more popular (it was much easier to
wash than the older woolen underclothes and so was likely
to be changed more often), and a public *attitude* toward
cleanliness developed, played a large part, but so did vacci-
nation and a host of other medical techniques. Hospitals
changed from places where if what caused you to go there
did not kill you, the infections you contracted during your
stay almost certainly would, to places where the benefits of
being there vastly outweighed the risks.

The conflict between the Galenic and the Spagyric physicians that had begun in the sixteenth century continued into
the twentieth, when the great pharmaceutical houses realized
that for them there was an immense advantage in chemical
medications. Unlike natural medicaments, they could be pat-
ented. The development of chemistry permitted laboratory

synthesis of many natural products. Not only could they be better standardized if made in this way but, being patentable, they could be the source of large amounts of money. A massive promotional effort was made by the new pharmaceutical houses to convince the general population that chemical products were superior to natural ones. This effort was largely successful. In the nation's medicine cabinets, herbs gave way to their synthetic correlates.

Since 1800, mainstream medicine has been based largely on an ancient idea known as the Doctrine of Contraries. The idea is so simple and obvious that it has come to be thought of as the most basic common sense. Anyone questioning it is thought to be simpleminded or fanatical.

The medical writer Brian Inglis described the doctrine simply: ". . . that where the body's working deviated from the normal, a counteracting procedure should be applied. Thus, a man suffering from constipation would be given a laxative; if he was feverish, ways would be found to cool him, and so on."

When germs were discovered to be implicated in many diseases, the idea seemed validated. If the germs were eliminated, the disease could be cured. If the patient experienced a deviation from the normal—the presence of specific bacteria—the physician had only to attack and destroy them and the disease would be cured.

This concept has certainly produced tremendous progress in many areas and has ended the threat of many disease. However, it has also blocked understanding of two major factors: first, the patient's own self-healing ability, and the fact that many symptoms (deviations from the normal) are the result of the restitutive attempts of the body—the Hippocratic *Ponos*. Second, that many patients with the bacteria present in their systems do not develop the disease; that the

"single-cause" concept of disease, although sometimes fruitful, is always false.

One reason that we retain the one-factor theory of disease (each disease is due to one factor, one germ, one virus,
and so on) is that it simplifies matters and makes problems
easier to deal with. And we human beings much prefer the
simpler explanations and approaches. In 1979 there was an
epidemic among the slum children of Naples, Italy, who began dying of a fulminating viral infection. Everyone agreed
that only those children living in the slums were dying. The
experts in Naples immediately got in touch with the Communicable Disease Center in Atlanta, Georgia, to initiate the
search for a vaccine. Think how this orientation simplifies
matters. You ignore the big question of why the virus does a
right about-face every time it comes to the edge of a slum
and stays away from children in the suburbs. You do not
have to worry about problems such as decent food and housing, breathable air, etc. Social problems are tough ones. The
idea that one virus equals one disease makes it possible to
ignore them.

(This is related to our insistent clinging to the mechanistic view of the universe. One reason we hang on to it—in the
face of a storm of contrary evidence—is that it is the simplest
and least mind-straining view of how things work that we
humans have ever developed. It may not be valid, at least for
large stretches of experience, but it *is* simple.)

The one-factor theory is gradually dying in medicine.
More and more physicians are coming to the viewpoint that
disease and health are problems not just of cells but of the
total human organism: that *people* contract disease and that
people must, therefore, be dealt with in resolving medical
and health problems. Typical of this new understanding is
the formation of such organizations as Physicians for Social
Responsibility sponsored by physicians of impeccable pres-

tige and position such as Helen Caldicott, Jerome Frank, Herbert Abrams, Sidney Alexander, and a host of others.

The fallacy of the "single-cause" premise has been shown in dramatic highlight by its inapplicability to many degenerative diseases. In spite of vast and very expensive research projects, *no single cause for these diseases has ever been found or is likely to be.* Farmers who have never smoked and who live in the clean air of the country do develop lung cancer; athletes who have very low cholesterol levels do have heart attacks; multiple sclerosis strikes apparently at random.

Wholistic medicine rejects the single-cause theory of disease. It is based on the belief that the patient must be seen as existing on many, equally important levels, and that steps should be taken against the disease *and* toward the development of health on as many of these levels as possible. Further, for each patient, an individual and unique combination of going "contrary" to the disease and of stimulating the patient's resistance to it and his growth toward health must be designed.

The idea that there is a natural remedy for each disease just waiting to be found has changed in this century, with a deep faith in science replacing the older faith in nature. Instead of hoping we might discover a specific plant or herb to cure each disease, we now waited, with firm conviction that it would happen, for the drug companies to develop an *artificial* substance that would be specific for each disease. Indeed, many such specifics were developed, including remedies for such conditions as amoebic dysentery, malaria, sleeping sickness, and blood poisoning.

One has only to read the accounts of the ancient chroniclers of the epidemics that ravaged their world to realize how much the sanitary revolution of the late nineteenth century, and the medical advances of the nineteenth and twentieth centuries, have contributed to our welfare. When we read about the hopelessness people felt as Athens, Rome, Byzantium, and the rest of the Classical and medieval worlds were ravaged again and again, how entire sections of the world were depopulated, how the course of history was changed by diseases with mysterious and terrible effects, we can begin to sense how far we have come.

The Byzantine historian Procopius described the great plague of the era of Justinian which started in A.D. 521.

> *During these times there was a pestilence, by which the whole human race came near to being annihilated. . . . For it did not come in a part of the world nor upon certain men, nor did it confine itself to any season of the year, so that from such circumstances it might be possible to find subtle explanations of a cause, but it embraced the entire world, and blighted the lives of all men, though differing from one another in a most marked degree, respecting neither sex nor age . . . it left neither island nor cave nor mountain ridge which had human inhabitants. . . . Death came in some cases immediately, in others after many days. . . . Indeed the whole matter may be stated thus, that no device was discovered by man to save himself, so that either by taking precautions he should not suffer, or that when the malady had assailed him he should get the better of it; but suffering came without warning. . . .*

So dramatic were the results of the new techniques for treating disease that the experiences which told the practicing physician that each patient was different in his susceptibility and his response to bacterial or other infection, or to any other disease process, came to be overlooked in medical training. Generation after generation of physicians graduated from medical school trained to look only at the specific disease, and not to be concerned with the ill patient. Individual differences among patients were largely forgotten, as were the patient's own self-healing abilities. Spurred on by the tremendous public prestige the medical profession had gained by its new skills, and by the belief that physicians had, or were developing in their laboratories, the skills finally to conquer disease altogether, medical schools ignored both the warnings of many outstanding experienced physicians about, and the actual hard evidence of, the limitations to their single-minded approach.

There were both warnings and contrary evidence in plentiful supply. Claude Bernard, one of the great medical researchers of the nineteenth century, wrote: "Illnesses, hover constantly about us, their seeds blown by the wind, but they do not set in the terrain unless the terrain is ready to receive them."

And Pasteur's last words were widely reported to be: "Bernard is right. The germ is nothing; the terrain all."

Around 1900 a number of English scientists drank glasses of cultures isolated from fatal cases of cholera. Tremendous numbers of cholera vibrios could be found in their stools; none developed true cholera. More recently American volunteers ingested dysentery bacilli under ideal conditions for infection (enteric capsules full of feces taken directly from people with bacillary dysentery were used) and very few developed the disease.

In the Lubeck Catastrophe of 1926, 249 babies were accidentally injected with tremendous doses of tuberculosis bacilli. Thirty-five percent died from acute TB, but sixty-five percent survived and were found to be free of disease twelve years later.

The epidemiologist Richard Doll has pointed out that even powerful carcinogenic agents do not necessarily cause cancer. There were 2,500 residents of Hiroshima and Nagasaki who were less than 1,100 meters from ground zero and survived. Less than 2 percent developed leukemia—a figure high enough to show the leukogenic effects of radiation, but low enough to show the importance of other factors.

Many individual physicians, often widely known and respected ones, saw the dangerous and self-limiting path medicine was on.

In 1927, Francis Peabody, president of the American Medical Association, wrote in a classic paper:

> *The most common criticism made at present by older practitioners is that young graduates have been taught a great deal about the mechanism of disease, but very little about the practice of medicine—or, to put it more bluntly—they are too "scientific" and do not know how to take care of patients.*

There was much dramatic evidence in the practice of every physician that each patient was different in susceptibility and in response to disease-causing agents. Sir William Osler, one of the greatest and most noted physicians of the early part of the twentieth century, said in a famous and often repeated statement: "It is more important to know what sort of patient has the disease than to know what sort of disease the patient has." But in spite of this evidence, and warnings to the contrary, the view that "one germ equals one disease," that each disease is caused *only* by a specific bacterium, became more entrenched. Individual differences among patients and the fact that there were restorative healing processes naturally inherent in the patient were lost sight of.

In the first half of the twentieth century, many medical people realized that the separation of mind and body in diagnosis and treatment had gone too far and was blocking further progress. Out of this realization came the modern field of wholistic medicine.

In *Tristram Shandy,* eighteenth-century novelist Laurence Sterne wrote: "Man's body and mind, with the utmost reverence to both I speak it, are exactly like a jerkin and a jerkin's lining; rumple the one and you rumple the other."

The theory of humors, which dominated the medieval and Renaissance periods, included a complex and sophisticated psychosomatic viewpoint. Until the seventeenth century, there was no real concept of the separation of mind and body. It was only after Descartes that this dualism was accepted. By the end of the nineteenth century, however, the separation had grown to a point that the interaction was not taught and was hardly mentioned in medical training or textbooks. The experience of all observant physicians that mental states affected bodily functioning was ignored.

It was left to the developing field of psychiatry, in the next fifty years, to recognize the crucial importance of this interaction in many diseases. Psychiatry, combined with advancing knowledge in the areas of physiology and internal medicine, made it clear to many physicians that they could no longer maintain the rigid lines of separation, that medicine and surgery could deal with specific disease and symptoms, but that the patient's emotional status would have to be changed if the condition were not to recur.

Typical of the best of the new approach is Martin Lipp's *Respectful Treatments: The Human Side of Medical Care.* In this manual for physicians, Lipp teaches expertly and lucidly how to deal with a patient as a full human being and how to avoid responding to him as a disease entity. He shows how the physician can be both disease specialist and health therapist. His patients are *respected* and are involved in their own medical decisions and treatment.

In his presidential address to the American Cancer Society in 1959, Eugene Pendergrass said:

> Anyone who has had extensive experience in the treatment of cancer is aware that there are great differences among patients . . . I personally have observed cancer patients who have undergone successful treatment and were living and well for years. Then an emotional stress, such as the death of a son in World War II, the infidelity of a daughter-in-law, or the burden of long unemployment, seem to have been precipitating factors in the reactivation of their disease which results in death . . . There is solid evidence that the course of disease in general is affected by emotional distress. . . . Thus, we, as doctors, may begin to emphasize treatment of the patient as a whole, as well as the disease from which the patient is suffering. We may learn how to influence general body systems, and through them modify the neoplasm which resides within the body.
>
> As we do go forward . . . searching for new means of influencing growth both within the cell and through systemic influences, it is my sincere hope that we can widen the quest to include the distinct possibility that within one's mind is a power capable of exerting forces which can either enhance or inhibit the progress of this disease.

The practitioners of the art of medicine have thus been in conflict over one issue since Roman times at least, and probably much earlier. Should medicine do as much, and as actively, as possible, or should it do as little as possible in order to deal most effectively with the disease? Should it be King Stork or King Log. Should the physician stress intervention and repair, or should he stress cooperation with the defenses of the body? Thanks to the tremendous and invaluable development of technology, medicine in the past hundred years has moved increasingly to the side of active intervention. We now *can* intervene far more and far more successfully than ever before. We have an *active* medical technique of great power for many diseases. But we are beginning to see the limitations of this approach and to understand that without the cooperation of the defenses and repair systems of the body, there are many things we cannot do. Much of the struggle and ferment in the field of medicine today results from this growing realization. We are beginning to comprehend that *the solution lies not in espousing one approach or the other, but in finding how best to combine them in a manner that is different for and appropriate to each patient.* This is what we mean by "wholistic medicine":

1. The patient exists on many levels and these are of equal importance.

2. Each patient is a unique individual and must be met and responded to as such. No person can be validly placed in a classification and then viewed as if the classification contained all that was important about him.

3. The patient should be actively and knowledgeably involved in his or her own treatment. The relationship between healer and patient should be one of mutual cooperation between two specialists with special and complementary bonds of information.

1

The poet and philosopher Goethe once wrote, "Nature has neither kernel nor shell." In this aphorism he was expressing the point of view we are discussing here. No one level of the individual, no *domain* is more important than any other. His chemical needs are as crucial as his interpersonal needs (but not more so) and these are as important as his spiritual needs. All are equally real and none can be validly reduced to any other. Wholistic medicine understands the fallacy of the "nothing but" idea: that to say a human being is "nothing but" nine dollars' worth of chemicals is a valid statement only if you plan to use him for fertilizer. Courage is not "nothing but" a reaction-formation to passive-dependent needs. Love is not "nothing but" an itching in the groin. A violin concerto is not "nothing but" the dragging of the hairs of a horse's tail over the guts of a cat. Religious feeling is not "nothing but" the fear of the dark. And conscious thought is not "nothing but" changing electrochemical states of the brain.

Just as psychology cannot be reduced to biology, so biology cannot be reduced to chemistry. Biological agents, for example, must be tested as such, not as chemical agents. (It is true that we must know their chemistry so that we can reproduce them and standardize them, but they behave quite differently as biological agents than they do as chemical agents.) To demonstrate this, we could use a rather extreme, but valid, example. I take a flask of water that is so chemically pure no chemical tests will reveal any impurities; none will reveal the presence of anything but water. From a chemical viewpoint it is completely inert. Then I spray it from an airplane over the state of Virginia and destroy the entire tobacco crop of the South. The water contains one molecule of tobacco mosaic virus. Chemically it is inert. Biologically it is a devastating bomb.

Pointing out that each domain must be understood in its own terms and not as a "reduction" of another domain, the psychiatrist Franz Alexander wrote: "It is hardly conceivable that the different moves of two chess players can ever be more clearly understood in biochemical or neuro-physiological than in psychological and logical terms."

Eugene Pendergrass, a past president of the American Cancer Society, has pointed out that the prognosis of cancer patients is very strongly affected by what happens in their personal lives. D. W. Smithers, past head of the British Cancer Council, reported the same experience. Neither of these physicians had had any psychiatric training or experience. However, they observed and related to their patients, and so saw what the nineteenth-century physician, not separated from his patients by an advanced technology, knew so well. A sizable scientific literature now exists clearly demonstrating the viewpoint of wholistic medicine: that the patient exists as a unique and complete person and must be medically evaluated and treated as such, and that all domains of his being interact. In short, that a person, not a group of cells, gets cancer, and that the person, not just his cells, must be evaluated and treated.

What the modern physician frequently forgets is that his actions exist in a context and cannot be meaningfully separated from it. The physician's attitude and beliefs and the patient's conscious and unconscious perception of them strongly affect the results of his medications and procedures. The patient's belief systems about the effectiveness of medical procedures affect how well they work. Since the physician is frequently enthusiastic about new medications, and the patient perceives this, the medications tend to work much better at first than they do later on. This is the reason for the old medical adage, "Use your new medicine while it still works."

In the sixteenth century, one of the most widely used cures for syphilis was guaiacum, and there were a great many attested cures. From the modern point of view, guaiacum is without value in the treatment of syphilis. Nevertheless, there is little doubt that in the sixteenth century it often was therapeutically effective. This is also true of a great many other medications and surgical procedures of the past. We can be certain that in the future many of our present widely used medications and surgical procedures will be viewed in the same way.

In wholistic medicine, we usually try not to use the term "levels of being" or "levels of the person" because this seems to imply that some levels are "higher" or "lower" or, "more real" than others. More often we speak of "aspects of the person," "realms of being," and so forth. Unfortunately there is a necessity conceptually to break up the person so that we can deal more effectively with the problems we face. In actuality, the person acts as a totality, but we simply do not have the language or concepts to deal effectively with this.

So we divide the person into "aspects," "realms," "categories," knowing that this is false to fact but necessary for the majority of us. The most usual and convenient division appears to be into "physical," "mental-emotional," and "spiritual." Other divisions are certainly as practical, but we in the West are used to this one.

By "physical" we mean those aspects of the person covered by nutrition, exercise patterns, and mainstream medicine. By "mental-emotional" we refer to those aspects usually covered and discussed in a psychotherapist's office.

The term "spiritual" is probably the most poorly defined in the English language, with many, many different meanings. In wholistic medicine we have had to adopt a definite meaning. This covers two kinds of activity. First there are those hard and disciplined kinds of prayer and meditation which lead us eventually to those moments of knowing that we are a part of the total universe and cannot be separated from it; that our feelings of loneliness and alienation are illusion. Whether one calls these moments "cosmic consciousness," "Christ consciousness," "satori," or any of the other names humanity has given them, does not matter. The second kind of activity comes from the fact that we are Westerners, not Easterners and in the West, those involved in spiritual development have always been more interested in what you did than in how you felt. St. John of the Cross wrote: "If you were in an ecstasy as deep as that of St. Paul, and a sick man needed a cup of soup, it were better for you that you returned from that ecstasy and brought him the soup for love's sake." And John Bunyan put it: "On the day of doom, men shall be judged by their fruits. On that day it shall not be asked if you believed, but were you a doer or just a talker." In our spiritual expression, it is necessary to demonstrate in work that we are concerned with more than just ourselves or our family. I have watched cancer patients who spend some of their free time working for peace organizations, ecology organizations, Big Brothers and Big Sisters, the Red Cross, and in their different and individual ways demonstrate this concern. I do not regard a patient with whom I work as finished with his development at this stage of his life until he has upgraded his life in all three spheres. The case histories at the end of this chapter will clarify ways specific individuals have done this.

## 2

Each patient is a unique individual and must be met and responded to as such.

*If you give the same nutrient to a patient with a fever and to a person in health, the patient's disease is aggravated by what adds strength to the healthy man.*
*—Hippocrates*

Hans Selye, who first developed the modern concept of "stress," presents three guidelines in *Stress Without Distress* for living fully amid the "wear and tear of everyday life" without illness or disease. The first of these guidelines is: "Find your own natural predilections and stress *level*. . . . Only through planned self-analysis can we establish what we really want; too many people suffer all their lives because they are too conservative to risk a radical change and break with tradition."

Today we are beginning to understand that individualized treatment programs are crucial for all the arts of medicine and healing. Anyone—nutritionist, physician, chiropractor, psychotherapist, psychic healer—who does not comprehend this, should be avoided like the plague he is.

The great teachers of mysticism have always understood that in psychic and spiritual development, there is a different path for each person.

In her autobiography, St. Therese of Lisieux wrote of the problems of being a spiritual director:

> *I know it seems easy to help souls, to make them love God above all, and to mold them according to His will. But actually, without His help it is easier to make the sun shine at night. One must banish one's own special tastes and personal ideas and guide souls along the special way Jesus indicates for them rather than along one's own particular way.*

When the Seer of Lublin was asked to name one general way to the service of God, he replied: "It is impossible to tell men the way they should take. For one way to serve God is through learning, another through prayer, another through fasting, and still another through eating. Everyone should carefully observe what way his heart draws him to, and then choose this way with all his strength."

In a similar vein, Rabbi Nachman of Bratislava wrote:

"God calls one man with a shout, one with a song, one with a whisper."

I recall a wise and expert psychoanalyst, Dr. Joseph Michaels, saying at a hospital psychiatric service staff conference, "I am prescribing the SNARIB treatment for this patient. It will do him far more good than psychotherapy or anything else in the pharmacy." He then turned to the physician who had presented the case and, asking him to make sure the treatment was carried out, left the conference room. Each of us, not having the faintest idea what this method consisted of, resolved to look it up immediately. When a library search failed to turn up a reference to a SNARIB treatment or even to a Dr. Snarib, we went back to Michaels as a group and asked him what he had been referring to. He told us that the term was an acronym for a method of treatment our medical and psychotherapeutic training had not prepared us for. It stood for "Skillful Neglect and Rest in Bed." Michaels then continued, "This is what *this* patient needs. He is a completely typical patient in that he is unique and what he needs is unique. Anytime you find two patients who need exactly the same treatment, you can be sure that the similarity is in your perception of them, not in them. And if you see more than two who need the identical treatment, it is quite likely that you are perceiving your own problem, not theirs, and prescribing for them what should be prescribed for you."

It is hard to overemphasize the importance of this point. So accustomed are we to believing that there is one right way to do things, that doctors tend automatically to slip into treating patients according to this concept. The belief is strengthened by long years of medical education emphasizing one cause for each disease and one correct procedure to follow in combating it.

We differ tremendously from each other in our genetic heritage, in our childhood and adult experience of the world, in the ways and degree to which we have nurtured or re-pressed our different needs, in the ways and degree to which we have directed our energies inward or outward, in our fears of ourselves and others, and in the meaning we have found for our lives. Knowledge of these differences is not just of theoretical interest, but is crucial at all levels for the treatment of disease and the search for health. One reason a trained anesthesiologist is required at every major surgical procedure is that each person differs in his response to an anesthetic and an expert is required to monitor the patient throughout the operation. A responsible physician who decides to prescribe a tranquilizer or other mind-influencing drug will not simply choose the most popular one in the general classification desirable, but will hand-tailor the prescription to the particular patient, and then will evaluate the patient's response at frequent intervals to see how this unique individual tolerates the medication. He knows that no two people respond to any chemical intervention the same way.

The psychiatrist Abraham Meyerson used to say, "As soon as you have decided, on the basis of theory and experience, that all patients who have 'A' also have 'B,' and that this can be absolutely depended on, you can be absolutely certain that within three days, a patient will come into your office with 'A' and not the slightest sign of 'B.' This will happen. The only question is will you be too blind to see it?"

A number of years ago I took a close relative to Mt. Sinai Hospital in New York City (a large teaching hospital with an excellent reputation) for major abdominal surgery. The drug of choice at the hospital for pain control during recovery was Demerol. This particular person did not respond to Demerol; for her it had no more effect than a sugar pill. I made sure that I told this both to the surgeon and to the anesthesiologist. For good measure (I *am* experienced with hospital rigidity), I saw that on her chart in large red letters was written "allergic to Demerol." (There are, by the way, a number of excellent and equally effective morphine-based drugs for pain control such as Dilaudid, Pantopon, or morphine itself.) After the surgery, in the recovery room, she was, of course, given a large dose of Demerol. She was eventually brought back to her hospital room on a stretcher, screaming in pain, with both blood pressure and temperature dangerously below normal and dropping. Since she had had a large dose of Demerol, nothing more could be given to her for some hours. The chief resident was called and was understandably concerned. He hovered in attendance, doing his best until the absolute minimum time was up. He then went to the floor's nursing station and came back with a loaded hypodermic, which he immediately injected. When after five minutes it had no effect, I asked him what it was. He replied, with surprise at my question, that of course it was Demerol, what they always used for severe postsurgical pain. This meant that she had to go through another three hours without pain relief, during which time she very nearly died. But for the happy fact that a couple of Delores Krieger's* expert and wholistically trained nurses had come by to see how she was doing, she would have. These nurses were able to get the patient through the next few hours of pain and raise her blood pressure and temperature by the use of breathing and movement exercises, meditation, autohypnosis, and psychic healing. They saved her life, but a basic flexibility of mind and openness to new experience (not to mention an attention to the patient's medical chart) on the part of the medical staff would have obviated the crisis in the first place.

---

* Delores Krieger is a professor of nursing at New York University Graduate School. She trains her nurses in an unusually wholistic approach to the patient at all levels of being from the chemical to the psychic.

In wholistic medicine, no two people can be treated the same. This is the reason that the only universally valid law in psychotherapy is Florence Miale's Law, which states that "any response of the therapist which comes from technique rather than human feeling is antitherapeutic." *Technique* refers to a stereotyped way of responding to *classifications* of people. If we treat people as if what is important about them is *only* the classification we have given them, we reduce them to less than they are, and so our response is antitherapeutic. The pattern of each person's life, and its possibility for expansion, is as different for each person as it is for each serious painting or piece of music.

St. Thomas Aquinas wrote in the *Summa*: "We do not offend God except by doing something contrary to our own good." There can be no contradiction in our caring for the physical and the emotional and spiritual elements of our being. As Aquinas knew so well, what is truly good for one of these elements of the gestalt that is our being is in essence positive for the others. He wrote: "God exercises care over every person on the basis of what is good for him. Now it is good for each person to attain this end, whereas it is bad for him to swerve away from his proper end."

The founder of the Hassidic spiritual development movement, the Ba'al Shem Tov, wrote:

> Since the beginning of creation no human being has been like any other. It is the task of each person to further this uniqueness, and it is the failure to fulfill this task which has held back the coming of the Messiah.

## 3

The patient should be actively and knowledgeably involved in his or her own treatment. One could not put it plainer or stronger than that.

*The patient has to participate in his own treatment. He must help himself to get well. Participation is more than taking a pill every day. He must choose a diet, exercise, relaxation, etc. Pretty soon you get patients who are no longer taking pills. . . . The miracle cure is when the patient helped cure himself. . . . It's more important what you don't do for a patient than what you do. . . . When a patient says, "What can I do to help?" you are in a new ball game.*

*—Marvin Meitus, M.D.*

The importance of patient participation in medical procedures is shown in the current acceptance of the "natural childbirth" movement and the role of the modern midwife. One of the most appealing aspects of midwifery is that it allows the mother—and where possible the father and often the whole family—to be a full and educated part of the birth process. The entire experience of birth is changed by a good midwife from a "thing" that is happening to the mother's body, and toward which she is passive (except for exhortations to "push"), to an integral part of the entire fabric of life in which the mother and father are active participants. A serious midwife has a good comprehension of the basic axioms of wholistic medicine. She sees the birth preparation process as one part of the total symphony of the family's life and tries to help the family see it in this way. She is constantly aware that the mother exists in many equally important domains, and is sensitive to, and refers to, specialists in nutrition, vitamin usage, exercise, psychotherapy, relationship needs, and spiritual concerns. She sees each patient as an individual who must be assessed, treated, and responded to as unique, and not as a member of a class of clients. She establishes a relationship with her clients as an equal rather than as an authority figure who acts out "mother knows best." Being a responsible practitioner of adjunctive medicine, she also works with medical supervision and emergency backup.

In the viewpoint of wholistic medicine, the patient must be involved as an active and equal partner. There are no *right* roads toward health, but only a best road for each individual. Since health is observable in the realm of consciousness, and in this realm there is only private access—only one person, the patient himself, can observe the data—the patient is as expert as the therapist. The patient knows the *ground* of his or her life, its color and texture, better than anyone else can. The therapist has a wider view and is more knowledgeable and experienced in many of the problems relating to health. Working together, they can form an effective and smoothly functioning team, but only the patient can judge how he feels or determine whether a procedure is helping or not. He alone is in the *midst* of his life and experiences it directly. Even gifted with the greatest possible empathy, the therapist is at a distance. In Goethe's words, "Gray are all your theories, but green the growing tree of life."

It is this respect for the patient, as a person and as the only real expert in how his or her own life is and feels, that is essential for the wholistic health specialist. If he or she cannot achieve this stance—as many cannot—they do not have the personality structure that will enable them to understand wholistic medicine or to function in it.

If a physician or other health provider is younger than you are and addresses you by your first name early in your relationship, beware! We prefer younger strangers—even if they are physicians—to address us as Miss, Ms., Mrs., or Mr. Doing so shows respect for us and not doing so shows quite the opposite. (I have known twenty-five-year-old interns to say to an older woman, "Hello, Mary. I am Dr. Smith" at their first meeting and have generally decided that such interns are probably not educable.)

The basic axioms of wholistic medicine are thus: if the patient is treated on all levels (for example, physical, mental-emotional, spiritual); if the patient is treated as a unique individual; and if the patient is encouraged to *participate* in the treatment as much as he or she is willing to do, then the patient's self-healing abilities are likely to be mobilized and brought to the aid of the medical protocol. This is the essence of this new approach to medicine that is rapidly gaining acceptance in the Western world.

The following case histories are illustrations of what we mean by Wholistic Medicine today.

T. WAS A very successful executive in his mid-forties. He worked for a large company, and had been promised a major promotion within a year. This was the job he had been aiming for since he first joined the company seventeen years before. He had been married for fifteen years to a chic, bright, and ambitious career woman. He described the marriage as "okay, no problems," and she concurred with this opinion. Both loved skiing and they took regular vacations in Switzerland. But the center of his world was his work, at which he was very good indeed. He was liked and admired by subordinates, colleagues, and superiors.

Two months before he was to move into the new job, a number of sudden symptoms brought him to seek medical help. A rapidly growing Hodgkin's disease (cancer of the lymphatic system) was diagnosed. At that time (the early

1960s) the prognosis for this condition was extremely poor, although it is now almost 85 percent curable. The Hodgkin's Institute in New York City had at that time no cases of five-year survival on record. T. was started on a radiation program. (This, with cortisone and nitrogen mustard treatment, was all that mainstream medicine had to offer at the time). During the course of treatment, he was referred to the staff psychologist as part of a research program then being conducted. After the exploratory interview, he told the psychologist that he felt his cancer "had something to do with, maybe was caused by, my emotions." (Thirty years ago the idea that it is fruitful to look at cancer as a disease of the whole organism, not as a set of problems of a group of cells —in short, that people get cancer and it is people who must be treated—was known to very few physicians, although a great many cancer patients were aware of it.)

The psychologist at the hospital where T. was being treated as an outpatient was experimenting with the health-therapist concept and, in this case, functioned in that role. T. began a program of psychotherapy. Encouraged to take his destiny into his own hands, he went to a nearby medical library and learned all he could about Hodgkin's disease. Not at all satisfied with what mainstream medicine had to offer, or with the extremely poor prognosis that was predicted for his condition, he decided to look further. He started by consulting an osteopath.

In most states, the O.D. degree is considered to be equal to the M.D., and the osteopath can prescribe and administer drugs and perform surgery when he or she believes they are indicated. The osteopathic physician places great emphasis on the self-healing abilities of the individual and on the "structure-function principle," which states that disease is usually a result of a displaced structure interfering with normal nerve and blood-system functioning. Osteopathy, therefore, stresses musculoskeletal manipulation, which often cures not only the structural problem (such as out-of-line vertebrae) but the corresponding functional or physiological problems as well.

The osteopath that T. saw recommended that he continue the radiation program prescribed by his oncologist and, in addition, prescribed a number of sessions of osteopathic manipulation. T. reported that the treatments made him feel a great deal better and that he had more energy after the series was completed.

It was hard at the time to find a nutritionist who had common sense, training, and experience with life-threatening diseases, but after some search T. managed to do so. He went on a strict vegetarian diet with heavy vitamin and mineral supplements. The diet was not one that would be recommended by most nutritionists today, but it seemed to be the best advice he could get at the time.

In addition, T. began to work daily with the Simonton technique, an adjunctive method of therapy specifically designed to stimulate his self-healing abilities and to bring them to the aid of the mainstream medical program. In this specialized meditation method one visualizes both the cancer cells and the self-defense forces in a concrete, "cartoon" fashion, and then concentrates on imagining a conflict between them, with the cancer cells being defeated. Thus one might (if this were the image one arrived at naturally, and which felt comfortable) visualize the healing forces as armored Crusader knights attacking and killing the cancer cells in the form of dragons. Originated by Carl Simonton, M.D. (who found that patients who did this meditation consistently while receiving radiation responded better than control groups who received only radiation), it has proved widely useful as an adjunctive method of cancer treatment. Physicians and others who teach this visualization method are now widely available, as are Simonton's book (*Getting Well Again*) and training cassettes.

During psychotherapy, it rapidly became apparent to T. that his marriage was an empty shell. Both he and his wife had settled for something very far from ideal. There was little to hold them together besides habit and T.'s belief (which his wife apparently shared) that nothing better was possible. He and his therapist explored T.'s deep despair about ever attaining any really loving relationship. At one point he said: "You know how it is, Doc, with a house with no insulation. No matter how much heat you put into it you can't get warm. You can only do that by having some of the heat reflected back at you. I always knew that that's how it was with me in life. No matter how hard I tried, no matter how much heat I put out, I would never be able to get warm." Working through and dissipating this despair, which stemmed from early childhood experiences, was a long and painful task.

When T. began to realize how little he had settled for in his marriage, he and his wife began to examine the situation together and—for the first time—to really talk about it. They went to a marriage counselor together and had several sessions with him. At the same time, T.'s wife was offered a better job that would require her moving to another city. This seemed to clinch it for both of them, and they divorced in an amiable manner. Both seemed to be quite relieved.

For a time after the divorce, T. felt that he wanted no relationships other than those in his work. He explored this feeling in his psychotherapeutic sessions, accepting and working through his underlying fear. He then began to date and saw a number of women a few times each. After about a year, one relationship developed into an affair and then a marriage. T.'s second wife is much more open and loving than the first. Reminded of his earlier remark about insulation, he grinned and said he felt "pretty warm now."

Through psychotherapeutic exploration of his work life, T. realized that the job he had been aiming at all those years now seemed to him to be a dead end. He felt that instead of producing the endless challenge and stimulation he had been fantasizing it would, the job probably would become boring in a year or two, like all the other jobs he'd had. After this new job, there would be no place to move to, and he would be "all dressed up with no place to go. Ever!"

When T. began to understand his feelings about work, he also began to see the fallacy of his presuppositions. The new job was one of which he could make anything he wanted, and his superiors were clearly hoping that he would be continuously creative and would develop in new ways. When he realized this, his despair over work also began to disappear. (T.'s despair over both his job and his emotional relationships, the feeling of being at a dead end in both, and the "sudden" appearance of a very severe disease, reminded the therapist of Jung's statement, "When an inner situation is not made conscious, it appears outside as fate." When he mentioned this during one session, T. thought about it for a very long minute, and nodded in complete and sad agreement.)

The therapist kept pointing out to him that he was doing beautifully in the spheres of his existence directly affected by the psychotherapeutic process, but that there were at least two other spheres he was neglecting—the physical and the spiritual. In the physical realm, the nutritional program was a beginning, but only that. Checking each time with his oncologist, T. began to experiment with a number of forms of physical activity. He joined a well-known New York athletic club offering a large number of activities and classes in everything from yoga to judo. He tried a number of these in an attempt to find one that felt right for this period of his life and that would help him with the necessary upgrading of his physical being. After trying several that were not relevant for him, he found that swimming laps in the local pool was exactly what he wanted. He would slowly swim dozens of laps with his mind focused only on the swimming, completely aware of what he was doing, not allowing himself to be distracted. He would generally emerge from the pool feeling slightly "high," "well put together," calm and energetic. He found that he wanted to do this four times a week before going to work and that the program was—at that point in his development—right for him.

Understanding (intellectually only at this point) that he was not expressing or nourishing the spiritual part of his nature, and that this was not permissible for him, not something from which he could escape, he began to try to discover and experience this part of himself. He knew he was searching for a larger context to his life and that this was expressed in different ways by different people: in some as a direct comprehension of their oneness with the cosmos; in some as an identification with the human race as a whole, working in a specific way for its development; and in some, ideally, as both. He attended several Catholic retreats and found them "interesting" and "pleasant," but with no real meaning for him. Some Zen seminars where the participants sat most of the day—in what for him, at least, was an uncomfortable position—he found interesting but not pleasant. After a number of experiments, he decided that the Eastern Breath Counting meditation described in Chapter 2 was what he was looking for, and he started doing this regularly one half-hour each day. He found that it made him feel better and more energetic all day, less "flappable," and more at home with himself and others.

As with the other disciplined meditations, this work

trains and tunes the mind as working in a gymnasium disciplines and tunes the body. If performed conscientiously and over a long period of time, it will also lead to transcendental understandings in which one begins to comprehend deeply our oneness with the entire cosmos and to *know* that our alienation and separation are illusions. Working regularly with a disciplined meditation program helps one function more efficiently in this world of the "many" and also in the world of the "One."

About a year after T. started working on the meditation program, he was invited by a colleague to attend a meeting of the American Association for the United Nations. He found that he responded to their approach and became interested in their work. He is now a senior officer in one of the chapters of this organization and is on several committees on the national level.

T.'s Hodgkin's disease responded well to the radiation program. The tumors regressed and did not reappear for about six months. A number of them then became apparent to X-ray and a further course of radiation was prescribed. The tumors again disappeared and have not reappeared in the thirty-odd years since.

T. has, in this time, changed both his exercise and his meditation program several times. What is right for us in one period of our development is not necessarily right in another. He has also changed his diet several times, both because of new information and because of his own needs. He worked at the job he was promoted to for about eight years and then moved to another company at a higher position. He enjoys his work. His marriage is a good one and he has two children, one of them an adopted Korean boy. He rates his life as "diverse, exciting, and fascinating. The only problem I have is that there are only twenty-four hours in a day and I have about thirty-six hours of things I like to do."

Here we see a pattern of individualized upgrading of life in as many domains as possible. T. took responsibility for his own life and sought help from as many teachers and therapists as he felt necessary. The wholistic approach does not mean using an adjunctive mode of treatment instead of mainstream medicine. (Although this is often the picture presented by those practitioners of adjunctive modalities who feel themselves to be in a power struggle with mainstream medicine. But these persons are fighting for control, not trying to establish a new approach to health.)

The wholistic approach to health is that it is far more than the absence of disease, it is a *process* of approaching one's fullest, most zestful, and joyful participation in every aspect of one's own life. The farther along one is on the path to this participation, the more one is using this method.

The following case history is included as an example of someone who, with no disease present, used this approach to life.

Martin was an associate professor of business management in a middle-sized college in a large East Coast city. He was in his late thirties and divorced. He had one child, who was in her early teens, lived with her mother, and saw Martin on occasional weekends and holidays.

There was nothing in particular wrong with him physically, but—as he put it later—"There was nothing particularly right with me or my life, either." He spent his vacations at singles' hotels in the mountains, which, as he described them, were "pleasantly promiscuous."

Martin had several single women friends and generally mild, rather friendly, long-term affairs with two of them. He would have four to six shorter affairs each year. These varied from a weekend to a month or two in length. He had no close men friends. He was witty and intelligent and was frequently invited to dinner parties by relatives or acquaintances who either needed an extra man for the evening or else had a woman friend or relative they wanted him to meet. He enjoyed these social events, but made sure that "they came to nothing." He had been once to a swingers' club that featured a nightly orgy, but had never returned. When questioned about this, he would tell the story of Voltaire, who had been invited to an orgy, accepted, acquitted himself magnificently, and refused to go again, saying, "Once a philosopher, twice a pervert."

When the fad was at its height, he took up jogging and did this several times a week. Later, in keeping with many in his social class, he switched to tennis.

In short—in the words Tolstoy used to describe the life of Ivan Ilych—"his life was most ordinary and therefore most terrible." It was pleasant, highly socially acceptable, busy, and essentially meaningless. He had found a way of life that made no demands on him and that was unrelated to his own particular being.

The summer he was thirty-nine he decided to take part of his vacation on a walking tour of New England instead of in his usual manner. (He recently had seen the original *Goodbye, Mr. Chips* on television, in which Robert Donat, leading a dull life as a teacher in an English preparatory school, meets Greer Garson on a walking tour of the Alps and this event changes his entire life. Martin later felt that this had influenced his decision.) Walking alone for three weeks, he began to feel that his life was somehow empty, that something was missing. Walking all day in the crisp spring air of Vermont and New Hampshire, he felt at once exhilarated and depressed. He knew he needed something new, but could form no idea of what that might be.

What he did not realize then was that he was going through what the psychiatrist Carl Jung called the "second adolescence." From Jung's viewpoint, those who are lucky enough to go through this generally do so between the ages of thirty-five and fifty. During the process, those who are able to succeed in the developmental task, find themselves shifting their primary orientation from concern with the opinions of others to concern with the growth of the self.

On his return to the city, Martin made an appointment with a psychiatrist he had met at a party, who had impressed him as "someone who seemed to be really anchored in the world." As they worked together, he began to realize that he had adjusted himself to life rather than the other way around. In the process he had completely lost sight of himself as an individual.

He began to explore with the therapist who *he* was. Among the first things he found out was that he was a person who enjoyed learning new things, but had "forgotten" this and had fed his mind no new nourishment for a long time. He began to read (and to audit some courses in his own and a nearby university) about the history of business management and its relationship to other aspects of cultural development. In two years, he found, rather to his surprise, that he was teaching several new courses (he had been teaching the same ones over and over for nearly fifteen years), that he had published several papers in his new area of interest, and had developed something of a reputation as an expert.

The exploration of his inner life led Martin to explore his deep fear of serious relationships and, indeed, of letting himself be deeply committed to anything. His relationship with his daughter improved markedly, as did his relationship with one of the two women with whom he'd had long-term relationships. They are now living together and both see it as a "probably permanent" arrangement.

He has rediscovered a college interest in jazz music of the twenties and thirties, and gets a good deal of enjoyment from it. He tried, at the therapist's suggestion, both Zen and yoga, but found they did not seem relevant to who he was and where he was in his development. He experimented with a number of physical approaches from karate to weight lifting and has finally found one, Tai-chi, that refreshes and invigorates him. Tai-chi is an ancient Chinese exercise system designed to integrate all the aspects of the person through a series of flowing movements on which the mind is completely focused. These movements, originally taken from the natural movements of animals and birds, appear to the observer as a dance of continuous postures set to the rhythm of slow, deep breathing. It is a movement meditation designed to use every muscle gently and to stimulate the circulation and the flow of energies in the body. It is both a physical exercise and a meditation. With practice it leads to a "passive exhilaration," a "calm excitement," and a sense of the unity of oneself and the universe.

On the wall over his therapist's desk there hung a sampler with the words, "If we heal the cosmos, we heal ourselves. If we heal ourselves, we heal the cosmos." Martin had gradually come to understand the need for *context* in his life; the need for participation in the human race. He now finds a great deal of satisfaction, and the easing of a need he did not earlier know was there, in working two evenings a week as the volunteer business manager of an ecology organization.

He is so engaged in and committed to his life that he does not ask himself much if he is enjoying it: he *knows* its meaning and value. He says with a laugh, "I wonder what my next walking trip will lead to."

As these two case histories illustrate, one of the cardinal principles of the new methodology is the requirement of activity on the part of the person involved. You must be active and seek for yourself. Find out what therapies are available and what are their likely results. It is relevant that the word "cure" derives from the same root as the word "curiosity." Be "curious" and take your destiny into your own hands. It is a lot safer there than in the hands of strangers.

There is a second principle that is repeatedly illustrated here: there are no basic contradictions between any methods that seek to upgrade various domains of your being. You do not do harm to one domain by doing good to another. As a specific example of this, Edward Cheraskin—one of the leading modern experts in wholistic health—has pointed out in a number of books and papers that there is no diet that is good for only one disease. A diet is either good for you or it is not. It is not good for your teeth and bad for your hemorrhoids or vice versa. If something is bad for your teeth, it is bad for the rest of you also. In his words: "The point being stressed is that common sense, if nothing else, would indeed suggest that if sugar is bad for the top of your body, it is equally bad for the bottom of your body. People do not walk around rotting from the waist up and healing from the waist down.

Cheraskin goes on to point out that a diet may be good for you or not good for you, but there is no one diet for everyone. Each person has individual needs. For example, if you live in a city (and therefore inhale a lot of lead) you need more vitamin C, which is a good chelating agent (an agent that unites with the lead and forms a substance that the body can excrete). If you smoke, or take aspirin, or are on the pill, you also need more, as these things interfere with your ability to metabolize vitamin C. If you do all four, you certainly need a lot more vitamin C than does a person whose lifestyle does not include these characteristics.

These principles—of the wholeness and unity of the person, and of the *uniqueness* of each person—are the basic tenets that underlie the field of wholistic medicine.

# About the Author

·

A psychotherapist and the author of twelve books including the bestselling *How to Meditate,* Dr. Lawrence LeShan is a pioneer in exploring the therapeutic implications of meditation. He has lectured throughout the United States and in Europe and has appeared on national television programs including "Good Morning America" and the "Today" show. He and his wife, Eda LeShan, divide their time between New York City and Massachusetts.